HEALTHY WEIGHT

HEALTHY WEIGHT

Simple Strategies for Successful Weight Management

YVONNE LONGMATEY

RN, CHC, MBA, BSN, BS

ParahBooks

Printed in the United States of America
Library of Congress Control Number: 2026903137

ISBN 978-1-7335660-1-8

Published by ParahBooks
a division of Parah Wellness
710 Dacula Road, Ste. 4A, #121
Dacula, GA 30019

www.ParahWellness.com

For everyone in pursuit of your
personal healthy weight,
this is for you!

CONTENTS

PREFACE

Yes, there is such a thing as "My Healthy Weight." It's the point where your health and weight goals meet, with YOU at the center.

Weight loss is often treated as a standalone goal. But lasting success comes when your weight goals align with your health goals. That's what this book is about: helping you find and maintain a Healthy Weight that supports your overall well-being.

Have you ever wondered why your weight fluctuates so often? This book will help you understand the reasons, and give you tools to manage it. Many people jump into diet programs without the right knowledge. These programs may work temporarily, but often at the cost of long-term health.

I've coached many individuals through the ups and downs of weight loss. And I've seen how a personal, health-centered approach makes all the difference.

Many readers of my previous book, *Healthy Me*, asked me to dive deeper into weight loss and share practical related health strategies. This book is my response. It is built on the principles of Healthy Weight and long-term success.

Before you start your next diet, read this book. Understand the key concepts. You are unique, and your weight loss journey should reflect that. This guide will help you make choices that support your health, not sacrifice it.

The right foundation leads to lasting results. It starts with knowledge. It starts here.

INTRODUCTION

Get YOU Back!
Real progress begins when
YOU become the focus again.

What does weight loss mean to you? Is it a distant dream you hope to reach someday? A bucket-list goal that fades quickly even if achieved? Are you struggling to manage and maintain your weight?

Jumping from one diet to another can be exhausting and frustrating. Why? Because YOU are often missing from the plan.

You're not alone. Many people chase a number on the scale, sacrificing too much in the process, sometimes even their health. But a Healthy Weight isn't just about numbers. It's about feeling great in your body and living well. It's personal. It's about your health, your lifestyle, and your goals.

To succeed, you need a weight management approach that puts YOU at the center. One that's responsible, effective, and sustainable. You should feel and look healthier after reaching your goals, not depleted or discouraged.

Science and research are always evolving, especially in nutrition and exercise. That's a good thing. It means better tools and insights to help you thrive. However, like a ship needs an anchor, you need a solid foundation. The right information helps you stay grounded, no matter how trends shift.

This book will help you build that foundation. You won't need to stress over whether to try Keto or go back to Atkins. You'll learn how to make choices that work for YOU. No gimmicks. No one-size-fits-all plans. Just practical, empowering strategies to help you smile about your Healthy Weight, and keep it.

Your journey starts now.

CHAPTER ONE

Your WHY

When you understand your "why," weight management stops being a struggle and becomes a meaningful, personal journey.

Have you ever tried to lose weight? Maybe that's why you're reading this book. Or perhaps you're looking to maintain a healthy weight, or even gain weight in a way that supports your health. Whatever your reason, one thing is certain: the right information makes all the difference.

Before we dive deeper, I want you to pause for a moment. Take a breath. Ask yourself this simple but powerful question:

"What motivates my desire to lose weight?"

Write your answer in a journal or notebook. You may want to revisit it as you read this book. That reflection will serve as your anchor, your reminder of why you started and what you're working toward.

People pursue weight loss for many reasons. Some are driven by health concerns, a diagnosis, a warning from a doctor, or a desire to prevent future illness. Others are motivated by appearance: wanting to look like someone they admire, fit into a favorite outfit, or feel more confident in their own skin. Some want to reclaim their energy, mobility, or sense of control. These reasons are all valid. They are personal. And they matter.

Your reason might fall into one of these categories, or it might be something entirely different. That's okay. What matters is that it's your reason. And like everyone else on this journey, you likely share one common goal: to feel accomplished when you reach your destination.

But here's where many people get stuck. They treat weight loss as a finish line. Once they hit their goal, they celebrate, and rightly so. Achieving a goal deserves recognition. But sometimes, that celebration turns into a long-term rampage. Boundaries disappear. Old habits creep back in. And before long, the progress fades.

This cycle of lose, celebrate, regain, is frustrating. It leads many to bounce between diets, plans, and programs, searching for something that sticks. But lasting success doesn't come from quick fixes. It comes from a shift in perspective.

So let me challenge you: instead of focusing on weight loss, focus on weight management. This is not a one-time event. It's a lifestyle. A mindset. A commitment to your health and well-being.

To succeed, you must see and accept your unique self. You have a personal, optimal weight range, not a single magic number. Your weight will naturally fluctuate throughout the day and week. That's normal. Factors like meals, hydration, sleep, stress, and even the time of day can affect the number on the scale.

Let me share a story that illustrates this beautifully.

While writing this chapter, my son, then a sixth grader, came to the dinner table with a big smile. "Mom," he said, "I weighed myself this morning." I smiled back, curious. He continued, "Then I weighed myself again after breakfast. I gained a pound!" He looked puzzled and asked, "Why did that happen?"

I explained that his breakfast was still in his stomach, it hadn't digested yet when he weighed himself the second time. It was simply sitting there, waiting to be processed. He laughed and said, "Wow, my stomach must be one serious bag!"

That moment stuck with me. It reminded me how easy it is to misinterpret the scale. A one-pound difference doesn't mean failure. It means your body is doing what it's supposed to do; digesting, absorbing, adjusting.

So here's a tip: weigh yourself at the same time each day when desired, preferably in the morning before eating or drinking. This consistency helps you track trends, not just numbers. And when you set your weight goals, think in terms of a range, not a fixed point. A narrow range allows for natural fluctuations without derailing your progress.

Now, let's talk about time.

Think of a pregnant woman. It takes her nine months to gain the weight associated with pregnancy. That weight is normal, expected, and healthy. Yet many women feel pressure to lose it within a week or two after giving birth. Why?

The truth is, most weight gain happens gradually, one choice at a time. A skipped workout here, an extra dessert there. These choices accumulate over months or years. So why expect to reverse them overnight?

I'm not saying it should take forever to lose weight. But I am saying it requires patience and self-kindness. Focus on making healthy choices consistently. Just like unhealthy habits add up, so do healthy ones. Over time, the right habits will help you lose weight, adjust to your new normal, and build confidence in your ability to sustain it.

This is the heart of weight management. It's not about punishing yourself or chasing perfection. It's about creating a lifestyle that supports your health, your goals, and your happiness.

A Healthy Weight helps you look and feel good. It reduces your risk of chronic illnesses like Type 2 Diabetes, heart disease, and joint problems. It supports your energy, your mood, and your quality of life. But here's the catch: many people lose weight and still develop health issues. Why? Because they neglected key factors nutrition, sleep, stress management and movement, in their pursuit of a number.

That's why this book emphasizes your personal healthy weight. Not someone else's. Not society's ideal. Yours.

To find it, you need the right information. You need strategies that work for your body, your lifestyle, and your goals. And you need patience, because real change takes time.

Wrap-Up: Key Takeaways

- **Know your "why."** Reflect on your motivation and keep it close.
- **Shift your mindset.** Focus on weight management, not just weight loss.
- **Understand your body.** Weight fluctuates; don't let the scale define your success.
- **Be consistent.** Weigh yourself at the same time daily and track trends.
- **Set a range.** Aim for a healthy weight range, not a fixed number.
- **Respect time.** Weight gain took time; weight loss will too.
- **Celebrate wisely.** Acknowledge your progress without losing your boundaries.
- **Prioritize health.** Your goal is to be healthy and at your ideal weight.

You've already taken the first step by picking up this book. That means you're ready. Ready to learn, grow, and take control of your health. This journey is about more than numbers, it's about YOU.

Let's move forward together. You've got this.

CHAPTER TWO

Understanding YOU

Your healthiest weight is not someone else's number. It's the place where your body, your life, and your well-being come into alignment.

For many years, weight loss strategies have focused on numbers, calories, pounds, BMI scores, while overlooking the most important factor: YOU. This numbers-first approach has led to frustration, confusion, and burnout for countless people. But after years of coaching, I've learned that the key to lasting success isn't found in a formula. It is found in the individual.

When YOU are at the center of your weight management journey, everything changes. Plans become personal. Goals become meaningful. And progress becomes sustainable. So before we go any further, let me remind you of something important:

You are unique.

There is no one else on earth exactly like you. Your body, your metabolism, your lifestyle, your preferences; they are all yours. That is why your weight is also unique to you. It's one of the reasons scientists have never been able to create a universal standard for weight. Every person is different, and that difference matters.

This uniqueness is especially important when it comes to understanding your Healthy Weight. It's not just about what the scale says. It's about how your body functions, how you feel, and how your weight supports your overall health.

Let's explore this idea further.

The Science Behind "Ideal Body Weight"

For centuries, researchers have tried to define an "Ideal Body Weight" (IBW). But it's proven difficult to generalize across populations. In 1964, Dr. G.J. Hamwi developed a formula to estimate IBW[1]. He accounted for differences between men and women, and even considered body frame size. His work laid the foundation for future formulas, including those by Robinson and colleagues in 1983[2, 3].

These formulas were originally designed to help calculate medication dosages. Over time, they've been adapted for broader use in nutrition and fitness. Today, many professionals use IBW estimates to guide their work with clients. But even the best formulas have limitations.

For example, the Hamwi formula doesn't account for lean muscle mass. That means it can underestimate IBW for muscular individuals. And while calculators make it easy to estimate IBW, it's still just that; an estimate, not a fixed truth.

So what does this mean for you?

It means that while IBW formulas can be helpful, they should be used with caution. They are a starting point, not a final answer. Your healthcare provider may use them to guide care, but they'll also consider your unique circumstances; your body composition, health history, and lifestyle.

Why Individual Factors Matter

Let's look at a real-world example. Children with Cystic Fibrosis, a genetic condition affecting the lungs, often have weight patterns that differ from typical growth charts[4]. Using standard IBW formulas for these children can be misleading, and even harmful. Their care requires a personalized approach that considers their unique needs.

This example highlights a broader truth: one-size-fits-all formulas don't work for everyone. That's why it's so important to understand your own body and work with professionals who respect your individuality.

You can explore tools like the ScyMed calculator, which uses the Hamwi method[5]. It's simple and widely used by healthcare providers. But remember, no calculator can capture everything about you. Use these tools as guides, not as definitions.

A Simpler Tool: Body Mass Index (BMI)

While IBW formulas are useful, I prefer a simpler tool for everyday use: Body Mass Index (BMI). It's easy to calculate and gives a quick snapshot of body fat distribution.

BMI is not a direct measure of body fat, but it offers a helpful estimate. It's calculated using the formula:

$$\text{BMI} = \text{Weight (kg)} / \text{Height (m)}^2$$

This ratio helps us understand how weight relates to height, and it's commonly used to assess risk for obesity-related conditions. The CDC offers a reliable BMI calculator[6]. Just note that BMI is interpreted differently for children and teens[7] [8], where age and gender play a role. In this book, we'll focus on BMI for adults.

BMI has its limitations. It doesn't distinguish between fat and muscle for example, but it is a practical tool for most people. It helps you personalize your definition of a Healthy Weight, and it's a great starting point for deeper conversations with your healthcare provider.

Personalizing Your Healthy Weight

Let's be clear: BMI alone should not be used to diagnose obesity. It's a screening tool, not a diagnostic one. Your provider will consider other factors including muscle mass and lifestyle habits, before making any conclusions.

But for our purposes, BMI helps us estimate fat distribution and understand how it relates to health. A tall person, for instance, will naturally carry more weight than a shorter person. That's normal. What matters is whether that weight supports your health and well-being.

So as you think about your Healthy Weight, remember:

- It's not about being skinny.
- It's not about fitting into someone else's ideal.
- It's about being healthy, energized, and confident in your body.

Both thin and overweight individuals can be unhealthy. It all depends on lifestyle choices, nutrition, movement, sleep, and stress. That's why this book focuses on Healthy Weight, not just weight.

Beyond the Numbers: Your Body's Story

Let's take a moment to reflect on how your body tells its story. Your weight is just one chapter. Other chapters include your energy levels, digestion, sleep quality, emotional well-being, and how your body responds to stress. These are all part of your health narrative.

When you begin to understand your body's signals, you can make better choices. You'll know when you're truly hungry versus emotionally eating. You'll recognize when your body needs rest versus when it's ready to move. This awareness is key to managing your weight in a way that feels natural and sustainable.

The Role of Professionals in Your Journey

Working with healthcare professionals on weight management can be incredibly helpful, when they see you as a whole person. The best practitioners ask questions, listen carefully, and tailor their advice to your unique needs. They don't just look at your BMI or IBW. They look at YOU.

So when you meet with a doctor, dietitian, or coach, don't hesitate to share your concerns, preferences, and goals. Your voice matters. The more they understand your lifestyle and values, the better they can support your journey.

Practical Tips for Applying What You've Learned

Here are a few ways to apply the insights from this chapter:

1. Calculate your BMI using a trusted tool like the CDC's calculator[6]. Use it as a reference, not a judgment.
2. Explore your IBW using the Hamwi method[5], but remember it's an estimate.
3. Track your trends, not just your numbers. Look at how your weight changes over time, and consider what might be influencing those changes.
4. Reflect on your habits. Are you eating in response to hunger, stress, boredom, or routine?
5. Talk to a professional. Share your goals and ask for personalized guidance.
6. Celebrate your uniqueness. Your body is not a problem to solve. It's a partner in your wellness journey.

Wrap-Up: Key Takeaways

Your wellness journey is personal. It's not about chasing numbers. It's about understanding your body and making choices that support your long-term health.

- **You are unique.** Your body, your weight, and your health are yours alone.

- **IBW formulas are helpful, but limited.** Use them as guides, not rules.
- **BMI is a practical tool.** It offers a quick estimate of body fat and health risk.
- **Personalize your goals.** Focus on what works for YOU, not what works for others.
- **Wellness is holistic.** It's about more than weight. It's about how you live, feel, and function.

You've already taken a powerful step by reading this chapter. You are learning to understand your body, honor your uniqueness, and build a foundation for lasting success.

So go ahead, calculate your BMI. Reflect on your numbers. And remember: this is just the beginning. Your Healthy Weight journey is about progress, not perfection.

Let's keep going. You've got this.

CHAPTER THREE

Getting Started

Your body tells a story no chart or calculator can capture. When you honor your uniqueness, weight management becomes clearer, calmer, and far more effective.

Starting a journey toward a Healthy Weight can feel overwhelming at first. But the truth is, getting started is often the most empowering step you'll take. It's the moment you shift from thinking about change to actually doing something about it. And the best part? You don't have to do it perfectly. You just have to begin.

This chapter is designed to help you take those first steps with clarity, confidence, and purpose. You'll learn how to track your progress, set realistic goals, and build habits that support long-term success. Let's begin with a simple but powerful action.

Action Item 1: Begin with Your Numbers

Grab a journal. This will be your personal space to record, reflect, and track your journey. Tomorrow morning, before breakfast, check your weight. If possible, check your height as well. Record both numbers in your journal along with the date.

Why morning? Because it's the time when your body is least influenced by food, drink, or daily activity. It gives you the most consistent and accurate reading. But if mornings don't work for you, choose a time that fits your routine, and stick with it. Consistency is key. Weighing yourself at the same time each day or week allows for fair comparisons and helps you spot meaningful trends.

Once you've recorded your weight and height, you're ready to calculate your Body Mass Index (BMI). Here's how:

1. Convert your weight to kilograms.
2. Convert your height to meters.
3. Square your height in meters.
4. Divide your weight in kilograms by your squared height.

That's your BMI for the day. You can also use the CDC's BMI calculator to verify your results[1]. Record your BMI in your journal along with your weight, height, and date.

Now, let's interpret your BMI using the CDC's adult guidelines[2]:

BMI	Weight Status
Below 18.5	Underweight
18.5 – 24.9	Normal or Healthy Weight
25.0 – 29.9	Overweight
30.0 & Above	Obese

Your goal is to fall within the 18.5–24.9 range. Notice that this is a range, not a fixed number. That's intentional. It allows for natural fluctuations of a pound or two, which are perfectly normal. So don't obsess over every decimal point. Instead, focus on making healthy choices consistently. That's what builds habits, and habits are the foundation of long-term success.

We'll talk more about habit-building in later chapters. For now, just know this: your quality of life matters more than any number on the scale. A Healthy Weight is about feeling good, living well, and enjoying your life, not just hitting a target.

Action Item 2: Set Your Goal

With your weight, height, and BMI recorded, it's time to set a goal. This is where many people stumble; not because they lack motivation, but because they don't set goals that are clear, realistic, and personal.

Let's change that.

Your weight goal should be:

- Relevant to YOU
- Specific
- Measurable
- Achievable
- Time-bound

Start by looking at your current BMI. Where does it fall in the CDC's guideline? If you're already in the healthy range, great! Your goal is to maintain it. If you're underweight, overweight, or obese, don't panic. You're not alone. And you're not stuck. Set a goal to move toward the healthy range, one step at a time.

If you have a health condition that affects your weight, consult your healthcare provider before setting your goal. They can help you choose a target that supports your overall wellness.

Let's break down the BMI formula again:

$$\text{BMI} = \text{Weight (kg)} / \text{Height (m)}^2$$

In this formula, your height is the denominator. For most adults, height remains constant. That means your weight, the numerator, is the key factor that influences your BMI. So, to move your BMI into the healthy range, you'll need to adjust your weight.

But remember: your healthy weight is unique to you. It's based on your height, body composition, and overall health. The weight that puts you in a healthy BMI range may be different from someone else's, and that's okay. Your goal is to find the weight that supports your health, not someone else's ideal.

Now, let's talk about time.

Weight loss takes time. It didn't take you a week to reach your current weight, and it won't take a week to change it. Be patient with yourself. Avoid obsessing over the process. Obsession leads to stress, and stress can sabotage your progress.

Instead, approach this journey with joy. Focus on building habits. Celebrate small wins. And give yourself grace on the hard days.

According to the CDC, a safe and sustainable goal is to lose 1–2 pounds per week[3]. If you're just starting out, aim for 1 pound per week. As you build habits and gain confidence, you may naturally progress to 2 pounds per week. The key is consistency, not speed.

Some days will be great. You'll make healthy choices, feel energized, and see progress. Other days may be challenging. That's normal. What matters is that you keep going. Over time, your good days will outweigh the tough ones, and your habits will become second nature.

Action Item 3: Journal Your Goals

Now that you've set your goal, it's time to write it down. This step is crucial. Writing your goals makes them real. It gives you something to refer back to, measure against, and revise as needed.

Here's what to include in your journal:

1. Your desired weight range. Use the healthy BMI range as a guide.

2. Your weight loss or gain goals. Be specific. If you're overweight or obese, aim to lose 1–2 pounds per week. If you're underweight, set a goal to gain weight gradually through nutritious eating.
3. Your timeline. Choose a time frame that feels realistic and achievable. This could be weekly, monthly, or quarterly.
4. Your motivation. Write down why this goal matters to you. What will it help you achieve? How will it improve your life?

Once your goals are written, you've officially started your journey. You've defined your destination. Now, you're ready to take the steps to get there.

And here's the best part: you can revise your goals anytime. As you learn more, grow stronger, and see results, your goals may shift. That's a good thing. It means you're evolving. You can update your goals monthly, every two months, or quarterly, whatever fits your lifestyle.

Wrap-Up: Key Takeaways

- **Start with your numbers.** Record your weight, height, and BMI in your journal for consistent tracking.
- **Use BMI as a guide.** Aim for the healthy range of 18.5–24.9, but remember it's a range, not a fixed number.
- **Set SMART goals.** Make them specific, measurable, achievable, relevant to **YOU**, and time-bound.
- **Focus on healthy habits.** Progress takes time. Avoid rushing and celebrate small wins.

- **Journal your goals.** Write down your desired weight range, timeline, and motivation to stay accountable.
- **Be patient and consistent.** Safe weight loss is about 1–2 pounds per week, according to the CDC[3].
- **Revise as you grow.** Update your goals as you learn and progress.

You've taken the first steps. You've recorded your numbers, set your goals, and committed to the journey. That's powerful. That's progress.

Remember, this isn't about perfection. It's about persistence. It's about showing up for yourself, day after day, with kindness and determination.

Your Healthy Weight journey is personal. It's not about fitting into a mold. It's about becoming the best version of YOU. And you're already on your way.

Let's keep going. You've got this.

CHAPTER FOUR

Weight and Health: The Right Way

You never have to sacrifice your health to reach your ideal weight. A Healthy Weight is where your ideal weight and your wellness meet.

Let's start with a truth that's often overlooked: it is absolutely possible to have a Healthy Weight. And not just a number on the scale that fits a chart, but a weight that reflects your best self. A Healthy Weight is your ideal weight, yes, but it's also a reflection of your overall wellness. It's a weight that supports your energy, your mood, your physical strength, and your emotional balance. It's a weight that helps you feel good, not just look good.

Too often, people chase weight loss without considering health. They cut calories, skip meals, and eliminate entire food groups. And while they may reach their target weight, they often do so at the expense of their well-being. Their bodies are depleted. Their energy is low. Their immune systems are compromised. Their moods are unstable. This is not the path to a Healthy Weight.

So let's redefine what it means to lose weight. Let's make health the priority, every time.

What Is a Healthy Weight, Really?

A Healthy Weight is more than a number. It's a state of balance. It's when your body is nourished, your mind is clear, and your spirit feels strong. It's when your weight supports, not sabotages your health.

Think of it this way: your Healthy Weight should help you feel energized, not exhausted. It should support your physical health, emotional stability, and mental clarity. It should allow you to move freely, sleep soundly, and live joyfully.

This is why I emphasize the word "healthy" in Healthy Weight. Because weight without health is just a number. And numbers alone don't tell the full story.

The Danger of Extreme Dieting

Many people work hard to reach their ideal weight, but in doing so, they give up key nutrients. They follow extreme diets that promise fast results but deliver long-term harm. They cut carbs, skip fats, and avoid entire food groups. And while they may lose weight, their bodies suffer.

Let's talk about why this happens.

Your body is a complex system. When it comes to nutrition, it operates in cycles: digesting food, absorbing nutrients, eliminating waste, and renewing cells. These cycles require fuel. And that fuel comes from the nutrients in your food.

When you deprive your body of essential nutrients, you disrupt these cycles as well. You force your body to pull resources from its own tissues and organs. For example, if you don't get enough calcium, your body may pull it from your bones, leading to joint pain and increased risk of fractures. If you don't get enough iron, you may develop anemia, leaving you tired, weak, and vulnerable to illness.

These effects aren't always immediate. Unlike holding your breath, which quickly leads to discomfort, nutrient deficiencies take time to show up. But make no mistake; they do show up. And when they do, they can be serious.

That's why it's so important to nourish your body every day. Not just with calories, but with nutrients. With vitamins, minerals, protein, fiber, and healthy fats. These are the building blocks of health. They support your immune system, your metabolism, your brain function, and your mood.

So when you're choosing a weight loss plan, ask yourself: Does this support my health? If the answer is no, it's time to reconsider.

Understanding Daily Nutrient Needs

Scientists estimate daily nutrient requirements using the % Daily Value (%DV). This tells you how much of a nutrient you need each day to support your body's functions. And here's the key: these needs are daily. You can't "stock up" on nutrients one day and skip them the next. Your body needs a steady supply.

Think of it like breathing. You wouldn't take one deep breath and then hold it for an hour. You breathe continuously, because your body needs oxygen constantly. The same is true for nutrients. You need them every day to keep your body running smoothly.

Let's look at a few examples:

- Calcium: Essential for bone health. If you don't get enough, your body may pull calcium from your bones, leading to pain and weakness.
- Iron: Needed for red blood cell production. A deficiency can cause anemia, fatigue, and poor concentration.
- Protein: Supports muscle repair, immune function, and hormone production. Too little can lead to muscle loss and weakened immunity.

These nutrients and many others, are vital to your health and sustenance. Cutting them out to lose weight is not a smart strategy. It's a short-term fix with long-term consequences.

The Risks of Popular Diets

Let's talk about two popular diets: Atkins and Keto.

The Atkins Diet was once a major trend. It emphasized high protein and low carbohydrates. Many people lost weight quickly, but some experienced side effects. Excess protein can lead to a buildup of uric acid, which may cause joint pain and kidney strain. I saw this firsthand in my coaching practice. People were losing weight, but they were also losing their health.

The Keto Diet is another trend. It focuses on high fat, moderate protein, and very low carbs. While it can be effective for some, it also carries risks. Long-term nutrient imbalances can affect liver and kidney function. And for some people, the lack of fiber and essential vitamins can lead to digestive issues and fatigue.

I'm not saying these diets are always harmful. But I am saying they require caution. They must be tailored to your individual needs, and monitored closely. And most importantly, they must support your overall wellness.

Balance and Moderation: The Winning Formula

In my coaching practice, I've developed a concept called Balance and Moderation. It's simple, but powerful. It means eating a variety of foods in appropriate portions. It means nourishing your body without depriving it. It means making choices that support both weight and wellness.

Here's how it works:

- Balance: Include all food groups: carbohydrates, proteins, fats, fruits, vegetables, and dairy. Each group offers unique benefits. Together, they create a complete picture of health.
- Moderation: Watch your portions. Eat mindfully. Enjoy treats occasionally, but don't overdo it. Listen to your body's hunger and fullness cues.

This approach helps people lose weight without sacrificing health. It helps them feel energized, not exhausted. It helps them build habits that last a lifetime.

And most importantly, it helps them enjoy the journey.

Wrap-Up: Key Takeaways

- **Healthy Weight is more than a number.** It reflects overall wellness: energy, strength, and emotional balance.
- **Avoid extreme dieting.** Cutting entire food groups or nutrients harms your body and long-term health.
- **Nourish daily.** Your body needs a steady supply of nutrients like calcium, iron, and protein to function well.
- **Be cautious with popular diets.** Atkins and Keto can work for some but may cause nutrient imbalances and health risks if not monitored.
- **Practice Balance and Moderation.** Include all food groups and watch portions to support both weight and wellness.
- **Choose sustainability over speed.** Quick fixes often lead to long-term harm; prioritize health every time.
- **You can have both.** Weight loss and health are not mutually exclusive. Commit to strategies that honor your body.

You don't have to choose between weight loss and health. You can have both. You can reach your ideal weight while feeling strong, vibrant, and well. You can nourish your body, protect your organs, and support your mind, all while shedding excess pounds.

It starts with understanding. With knowledge. With a commitment to doing things the right way, not the fast way.

So let's make a promise. Let's commit to putting Healthy and Weight together every time. Let's stop chasing numbers and start building wellness. Let's choose balance, moderation, and nourishment. Let's honor our bodies and support our health.

Because you deserve to feel good. You deserve to live well. And you deserve a Healthy Weight that reflects your best self.

Keep moving forward with intention and confidence. You've got this!

CHAPTER FIVE

Eat and Lose: ABCs of Healthy Nutrition

You don't have to starve to lose weight; you just need a strategy that nourishes your body and supports your goals. The ABCs of Healthy Nutrition show you how to make every bite count.

Let's talk about something powerful: the idea that you can eat and still lose weight. Not only is it possible, it's the most sustainable way to reach and maintain your Healthy Weight. But to do it right, you need more than just a meal plan or a calorie tracker. You need a foundation. You need a mindset. You need a system that puts YOU at the center.

In this chapter, I'll walk you through the **ABCs of Healthy Nutrition**, a simple but powerful framework that will help you make smart choices and build lasting habits:

- **A – Awareness**: Know what you're eating and why. Understand your body's needs and how food meets them.
- **B – Balance**: Learn to balance nutrients and calories. Avoid extremes. Choose variety and moderation.
- **C – Consistency**: Build habits that last. Make healthy eating a lifestyle, not a temporary fix.

These ABCs are not just concepts; they are your compass. They'll help you navigate the confusing world of nutrition and make choices that support your health, your goals, and your life.

Let's walk through each one together.

A – Awareness: Know What You're Eating

Awareness is the first step. You can't change what you don't understand. And when it comes to food, most of us are operating on autopilot. We eat what's convenient, what's familiar, or what's marketed to us. Rarely do we pause and ask, "What does my body actually need right now?"

Let me share a quick story.

Years ago, I was coaching a client who had tried every diet under the sun. Keto, Paleo, Atkins, you name it. She was frustrated, exhausted, and confused. When I asked her what she ate in a typical day, she rattled off a list of foods. But when I asked why she chose those foods, she paused. "I don't know," she said. "I guess I thought they were healthy."

That moment was a turning point. We started focusing not just on what she ate, but why. We looked at labels, nutrients, and how her body responded to food. She began to notice patterns; foods that made her feel energized, foods that made her sluggish, and foods that triggered cravings. That awareness changed everything.

So here's your first challenge: start paying attention. Look at your plate. Ask yourself:

- What nutrients am I getting?
- How does this food make me feel?
- Am I eating out of hunger, habit, or emotion?

This isn't about judgment; it's about curiosity. The more you understand your food, the more empowered you become.

In food and weight management, the easiest approach is to focus on calories. That is what most people do. Yes, by all means, do that because this is a major influence on weight gain, loss, or maintenance. But only focusing on calories can harm long-term health. A better way to do this is to first analyze the nutrition of what you eat. Then follow this with your calorie count. This approach will help put you at the center of your weight management goals. This method lets you first think about your body's needs. Then, consider how to meet them while managing your weight. This approach is very effective for long-term weight and health.

This strategy to weight management will help you know your wellness needs and how to meet them. This gives you a strong sense of motivation. It also affects your choices for years to come. This approach can help you avoid problems. It prevents today's choices from depriving you of what you need tomorrow. Poor decisions would negatively affect your health. It all boils down to this: Know your body's needs. Then, fit them within your daily calorie limits. This is key to effective weight management.

Knowing what you need is where the confusion lies for most people. It can begin to get complicated if you do not have a solid overview of the basics. I will stick to the essential basics. This way, you can analyze everything else you learn with the right perspective. Winds can pull down the structure of a building when the foundation is weak. Unfortunately, this foundation is not in place for most people. Because of this, most people fail at successful weight management. They hop from diet to diet and can't manage their weight. I want to give you the right building blocks. Then, you can view your next meal with a healthy perspective. Additionally, with a solid grasp of these basics, you will be able to tweak any dietary regimen to fit your needs.

B – Balance: Nourish Without Neglect

Balance is the heart of healthy eating. It's about giving your body what it needs, without going overboard. It's about choosing foods that fuel you, not just fill you.

Let's explore the five major food groups and how they support the ABCs of nutrition.

The Five Major Food Groups

1. Fruits and Vegetables
2. Grains
3. Protein
4. Dairy
5. Fats and Oils

Each group plays a unique role in your health. Understanding these roles will help you build meals that nourish your body and support your weight goals.

Fruits and Vegetables: The Bedrock of Wellness

Let's begin with one of the most essential but often overlooked parts of the Food Pyramid: fruits and vegetables. Their role may seem subtle, but they are foundational to wellness and successful weight management.

Unlike other sections of the pyramid that have evolved in name, description, and serving size, fruits and vegetables have remained largely unchanged. While some global food pyramids rearrange them for different dietary models, their importance remains constant, even as nutrition science evolves.

I call them the *bedrock* of smart food choices. When fruits and vegetables are rightfully placed in your diet, they bring joy to your meals and support your health. And that word *rightfully*, is key. This is where YOU come in. Your preferences should guide how you include them. When your choices reflect your tastes and lifestyle, you're more likely to stay consistent. And consistency is the cornerstone of effective weight management.

YOU are essential to your success. Many weight management strategies focus on rigid diet plans and strict regimens, often leaving YOU out of the equation. This can lead to frustration and fluctuating weight patterns that follow the latest trends rather than your personal needs.

Let's take a different approach; one that puts YOU at the center. This empowers you to create a plan that works for you and supports long-term wellness.

Fruits and vegetables are rich in vitamins, minerals, and plant-based nutrients called *phytonutrients*, which play a vital role in boosting health. Some vegetables, like lettuce, are very low in calories but high in phytonutrients. Vegetables generally fall into five categories:

- Starchy (e.g., sweet potatoes)
- Dark green
- Red & orange
- Legumes (beans & peas)
- Other vegetables

Starchy vegetables tend to be higher in calories but still offer valuable nutrients. Legumes provide a modest amount of protein, more than other vegetables, though less than animal sources; they also come with their own unique phytonutrients. Colorful fruits and vegetables are especially rich in phytonutrients. Sweeter fruits contain natural sugars, which increase their carbohydrate content along with their phytonutrient value.

Understanding these facts help you analyze your meals more effectively. The sweeter the fruit or the starchier the vegetable, the more carbohydrates it contains including natural sugars, along with its phytonutrients. Whenever possible, eat fruits and vegetables in their whole forms. They are excellent sources of fiber and phytonutrients, which help you feel full and satisfied, an important strategy for managing weight.

As we move forward, I'll build on these insights. For now, remember: fruits and vegetables are packed with vitamins and minerals. Eat plenty of them, and aim for variety. A strong start to healthy weight management begins with knowing this part of the pyramid well. Train yourself to include them in meals and snacks. Be creative! This will help YOU get enough each day.

The key takeaway? Fruits and vegetables are essential players. They should always have a place on your plate, whether snacks or main meals.

I encourage you to take a thoughtful look at this food group based on what we've discussed. This is a crucial step toward achieving and maintaining a healthy weight. Soon, I'll explain why, and how you can rearrange your personal pyramid to better meet your wellness needs. We'll explore that when we reach the stage of putting it all together.

Grains: Energy with Intention

This is another major part of the Food Pyramid. Over the years, its components and labels have evolved. What we now call the *grains* section was once broadly referred to as *carbohydrates*. Unfortunately, during that time, many people consumed excessive amounts of refined carbs, contributing to a decline in population health. A high intake of refined carbohydrates may have played a role in the rise of obesity. Even today, this section is sometimes still referred to as the *carbohydrate group*.

I like to call this group *energy boosters*, and yes, that includes the quick ones. Carbohydrates break down into simple sugars like glucose, which the body uses for energy. That's why many energy drinks are loaded with sugar. Athletes, for example, often rely on these sugary drinks for a fast energy boost during competition. They've learned how to use carbohydrates strategically for on-demand energy.

But for everyday wellness and weight management, it's important to make smart carbohydrate choices. Your goal should be to fuel your body, not just quickly, but steadily. Aim for a slow, sustained release of energy from the foods you eat. To do this, choose complex carbohydrates over refined ones. Starchy whole vegetables are a great place to start.

Refined carbs release energy rapidly, which can overwhelm your body. Your systems work hard to process this quick energy, but over time, that constant strain can lead to exhaustion. Foods and drinks high in refined sugars create this cycle: a quick spike in energy, followed by a crash. That's why it's best to consume them in minimal amounts.

Of course, there are exceptions. People with diabetes may need quick-sugar sources to raise blood sugar levels when necessary. Athletes may use refined carbs for a performance boost. But for most people, especially when managing weight, the goal should be to choose carbohydrates that retain their complex form, the least processed options available.

Think of the produce section at your grocery store. The closer a food is to its natural state, from farm to plate, the better it is for your health. That is why the produce section is one of the best places to shop for your weekly meals.

Try to limit foods that have undergone extensive processing. Pickled items, chips, and similar snacks fall into this category. You don't have to eliminate them entirely; just enjoy them occasionally and in small amounts. When shopping outside the produce section, look for whole grain options, especially if you enjoy bread or crackers.

When planning meals and snacks, focus on carbohydrates that are high in fiber. Fiber slows digestion, helping to sustain energy levels and keep you feeling full. That's a powerful tool for effective weight management.

So, when you think of carbohydrates, think *energy*. That energy can be quick or sustained, depending on your choices. For wellness and weight goals, choose complex carbs that provide lasting energy. Refined carbs, especially when eaten alone, digest quickly. They may give you a burst of energy, but they lack nutrition and won't keep you full. Many also contain preservatives and other additives your body doesn't need.

When you eat more refined carbs to satisfy hunger, your body stores the excess calories as fat. Hunger is your body's way of asking for fuel, it's your job to respond with the right kind of fuel. There's an efficient way to do this, and I'll show you how. It will help you stay on track with your weight and wellness goals.

We'll bring it all together; how to manage your plate, your snacks, and your energy, in a later chapter.

Protein: The Builder and Sustainer

Protein is another major food group, and an essential part of a healthy diet. This category includes meats, poultry, fish, and eggs as primary sources. Legumes, such as beans and peas, also provide protein. Interestingly, legumes are part of both the protein and vegetable groups, depending on how they're categorized. They offer a low to moderate amount of protein, depending on how much you eat.

That said, don't skip adding other vegetables to your plate just because you've included legumes. Like legumes, nuts are another flexible food; they can also fall into multiple categories. They also provide low to moderate protein, and contain healthy oils, which we'll explore more in the *Fats and Oils* section.

Proteins are the building blocks of your body. They help form muscles, bones, tissues, and cartilage. Even your blood is made up of connective tissue which is primarily built from proteins. That's why bodybuilders often consume high-protein diets and protein shakes. These shakes typically include protein along with sugars, vitamins, and minerals to support muscle growth.

Your body also uses protein to produce hormones and enzymes, both of which are essential for healthy functioning. In short, adequate protein intake is vital for your health and wellness.

As you age, especially after 50, it's important to eat a variety of proteins in moderation. This can help prevent joint pain caused by excess uric acid, a byproduct of purines found in certain protein-rich foods. For some people, high uric acid levels lead to gout, which causes painful joint swelling. In many cases, simply normalizing protein intake can help alleviate these symptoms.

For adults, a helpful visual for portion size is the size of a deck of cards or the palm of your hand when serving meat or fish. These simple cues help you meet your body's needs without overdoing it.

For growing kids and teens, protein is especially important for healthy development. It's also helpful to monitor the intake of other food groups to ensure balanced nutrition.

When you think of protein, remember its critical role: it supports the formation, repair, and maintenance of body tissues, and it's essential for producing hormones and enzymes that keep your body running smoothly.

Aim for reasonable servings of protein. The general recommendation is about 0.36 grams per pound of body weight. For athletes, coaches often suggest 0.5 to 0.8 grams per pound to support muscle building. Individual needs would vary. For example, a sedentary woman of average weight needs about 46 grams of protein daily, while a sedentary man needs about 56 grams. Just like athletes, your body needs the right fuel to compete in life.

Eating enough protein also helps you feel full longer, which can reduce the temptation to overeat or reach for empty-calorie foods. Nuts, legumes (like beans), and dairy products are great sources to help you meet your daily protein needs. Just remember, more isn't always better. The right amount is what your body needs.

Now, let's talk about snacks. If you're feeling hungry between meals, try adding a few nuts or a serving of dairy. Combine them with fruits, vegetables, or whole-grain crackers. This gives you a satisfying mix of protein, fiber, and healthy fats; a powerful trio to keep you full and energized.

Here's a practical tip: based on what you've learned so far, start listing some healthy, weight-maintaining snacks that you enjoy. As we continue, you'll be able to compare your choices with your health goals and make adjustments as needed. This is how you build a personal plan that works for YOU.

Dairy: Bone Health and Beyond

The dairy section of the Food Pyramid has sparked debate for years. Some people are allergic to dairy products, and for them, it's essential to avoid these foods entirely. For others, the challenge lies in understanding how dairy affects their health. Based on extensive research and personal experience, I've found a helpful way to navigate this: the concept of *benefits versus disadvantages.* Let's apply that to dairy so you can make informed, personal choices.

If dairy is a good fit for you, it offers many benefits. Starting your day with a glass of milk, for example, can positively impact your health. Dairy products are rich in calcium and vitamin D, and they also provide protein, vitamin A, phosphorus, and vitamin B12. These nutrients help you meet your daily intake goals and support your body's essential functions.

The dairy category includes milk and related products, but only those that retain their calcium content. Products like butter, which lose calcium during processing, don't qualify. Always read product labels when shopping. Most dairy items provide 15–25% of your daily calcium needs, depending on portion size. This category includes cheese and yogurt as key items. Fermented dairy products like yogurt are especially valuable; they are a major source of beneficial bacteria that support gut health.

Dairy is important because it contains both calcium and vitamin D. Vitamin D helps your body absorb calcium, making this combination especially powerful. Your bones form the framework that supports your body; they deserve care and attention. Poor bone health can affect both children and adults, often leading to preventable injuries and fractures. You can strengthen your bones by being mindful of your calcium intake, and dairy can help you do that.

If you're allergic to dairy, turn to green leafy vegetables and their relatives, like broccoli. These are excellent sources of calcium. If you're not allergic, include both dairy and leafy greens in your diet. This balanced approach helps you get the most out of dairy while consuming it in moderation.

Let's pause here to highlight vitamin B12, because it plays a vital role in your health. It's an essential coenzyme involved in metabolism, red blood cell formation, and nerve function. Red blood cells are crucial. They transport nutrients and oxygen and help remove waste and carbon dioxide from your tissues and organs. Healthy cellular metabolism supports effective weight management.

You can get this essential nutrient vitamin B12, from animal products. Poultry, meat, fish, milk and milk products, and eggs are all excellent sources. In its natural state, vitamin B12 is bound to protein. During digestion, stomach acids release it from the protein. Once free, it binds to a special protein called *intrinsic factor*, produced in the stomach. This complex is then absorbed and transported into the bloodstream.

Some foods, like cereals, are fortified with vitamin B12 during processing. Most people who consume animal proteins and fortified foods get enough of this nutrient. However, some individuals have absorption issues due to digestive conditions. A simple test at your doctor's office can identify such challenges. In those cases, supplements or B12 injections may be necessary.

A deficiency in vitamin B12 can leave you feeling sluggish, lightheaded, or lethargic. It may also cause loss of appetite, constipation, or diarrhea. Over time, the nervous system can be affected, leading to symptoms like muscle weakness, tingling, or numbness. Many nutritional deficiencies show up in the body through symptoms. Eating a balanced diet supports your health and helps you and your doctor identify concerns more quickly and accurately.

Dairy products can help you meet your daily vitamin B12 needs[1]. This nutrient is vital for cellular metabolism and weight management. The recommended daily intake for adults is between 2.4 mcg and 2.8 mcg[2]. Some studies suggest that milk drinkers experience several health benefits[3].

That said, milk isn't for everyone. Some studies show it may cause issues for some people, as in those who are lactose intolerant. People who are lactose intolerant may have safer dairy options if desired. Shop to suit your needs and preferences. There are also myths that discourage people from enjoying milk's benefits. One common belief is that milk increases mucus production in the respiratory tract. I used to believe that too, until I did the research. Let me gently challenge that idea if you hold it as well.

Milk thickens saliva, which can make swallowing feel harder, but it does not increase mucus production[4].

Still, if milk causes discomfort, it's wise to proceed with caution. Everyone's body responds differently to foods, and dairy is no exception. Pay attention to how your body reacts, especially when you have colds or coughs. This awareness will help you enjoy milk in a way that supports your health.

If you choose to include milk in your diet, you can enjoy its benefits while minimizing drawbacks. Quality matters. Opt for dairy products from animals not treated with hormones. Over the years, I've found that the benefits of dairy far outweigh the drawbacks, especially when consumed in moderation. Many people run into issues simply because they consume too much. Even good things can become harmful in excess. If needed, take a break from dairy for a season to reset.

Moderation is a powerful concept. It allows you to enjoy milk's benefits while reducing its downsides. Use research wisely, and always put YOU at the center of your decisions. Research offers valuable insights, but when taken out of context, it can lead to confusion. Stay focused on the big picture and how it applies to your unique needs.

Dairy can support weight management when consumed in moderation. If your goal is to gain weight, whole milk products may be helpful. If your goal is to lose or maintain weight, choose 2% or skim milk options. And while you're at it, watch the sugar content. Choose unsweetened varieties most of the time, and save sweetened options for dessert moments. Personally,

I prefer 2% milk, it's close in taste to whole milk but with fewer calories.

Dairy also provides protein, which supports satiety and weight control. When you think of dairy, think bone health, vitamin D, and calcium, a trio that works together. Vitamin D helps your body absorb calcium, and both are essential for strong bones and overall wellness. Drinking milk in the morning may even boost cellular metabolism, thanks to its vitamin B12 content. This can help your cells function more efficiently, breaking down nutrients instead of storing excess fat. I'll expand more on this idea of *arming your cells* for better performance later in the book. It's a key part of healthy weight management.

The recommended dairy intake is 2–3 servings per day. This is how I apply moderation: I usually start my day with milk and a low-sugar, healthy cereal. I also take 300 mg of calcium with vitamin D alongside my milk. This mimics the way nutrients are absorbed from food and enhances absorption of the supplement. That's two servings done early in the day. I then aim to get more calcium and vitamin D from leafy greens and healthy snacks. This approach lets me enjoy occasional dairy-based snacks, guilt-free. When I do, I stay mindful of the calories and adjust my meals later in the day or week if needed.

I'm not a heavy dairy consumer, but practicing moderation helps me benefit from different schools of thought. I check in with my doctor regularly and review my blood work to ensure my habits support my health goals. I look for healthy levels of vitamin D and calcium in my bloodstream. I also listen to my body. When my bones feel strong and supported, I know I'm on the right track. You can try this approach too.

For children and young adults, it's best to get calcium from food rather than supplements. The small amounts in multivitamins are usually enough. In some cases, a pediatrician may recommend a calcium or vitamin D supplement, but this should be monitored by a healthcare provider. Remember, the body absorbs nutrients best from food.

I began supplementing after the birth of my first child. I was breastfeeding and couldn't meet my calcium and vitamin D needs through food alone. I started experiencing joint pain, and even climbing stairs became difficult. After analyzing my routine, I realized my low intake of calcium-rich foods was affecting my bones. My body was pulling calcium from my bones to support breastfeeding. A small calcium and vitamin D supplement helped resolve the issue quickly.

Over time, I've adjusted my supplement intake to match my needs. Like anything else, excess can cause problems, so I only take a small amount and get the rest from food.

I hope sharing what works for me gives you a helpful starting point. Experiment to find what works for YOU. If your body doesn't tolerate dairy, there are plenty of other options. The key is to make choices based on your own experience, not someone else's. Focus on managing your weight in a way that supports your overall wellness.

Fats and Oils: Choose Wisely and Strategically

Fats play a key role in both wellness and weight management. When it comes to fats and oils, your body needs small to moderate amounts, but they must be the right kinds. The healthiest fats come from foods rich in monounsaturated and polyunsaturated fats. These are primarily found in plant-based foods like seeds, nuts, and avocados, as well as in fatty fish such as salmon, mackerel, and sardines.

These "good fats" support your health in powerful ways. Cholesterol tests at your doctor's office measure both "good" and "bad" fats. HDL (High-Density Lipoprotein) reflect your "good cholesterol" levels. Monounsaturated fats support levels of "good cholesterol". They are liquid at room temperature but start to solidify when chilled. You'll find them in avocados, peanuts, and olive oil. These are among the most preferred fats. Polyunsaturated fats are also "good fats". They remain liquid even when refrigerated. They're found mostly in fatty fish, plant-based oils, seeds and nuts.

These fats are especially beneficial for your brain and heart health. They nourish your body and support vital organs. That's why I call them "good fats."

On the flip side are the "bad fats," reflected in your LDL (Low-Density Lipoprotein) levels. These are primarily saturated fats, found in animal products. To reduce your intake of bad fats, trim visible fat from meats and remove the skin from poultry. Also, limit your consumption of deep-fried foods. It takes intentional effort to increase your intake of good fats while reducing the bad.

The good news? Your body only needs small to moderate amounts of good fats. And I'll soon show you a simple, strategic way to include them. Keep in mind that fats are calorie-dense: one gram of fat contains nine calories, while carbs and protein each contain four calories per gram. So even small amounts of good fats can make a big impact on your health and weight goals.

When you think of fats, think plants and fish. These sources are good for your heart, brain, and overall wellness. Aim to keep saturated fat intake below 10% of your daily calories.

Now let's talk about trans fats, the worst type of fat you can consume. Trans fats come in two forms: naturally occurring and artificial. Natural trans fats are found in small amounts in fatty meats and dairy. Artificial trans fats are created through a process called partial hydrogenation, where hydrogen is added to liquid oils to make them solid.

Food manufacturers often use partially hydrogenated oils because they're inexpensive and improve shelf life, texture, and stability. Unfortunately, they're found in many common foods like fast food, frozen pizzas, baked goods, margarine, creamers, spreads, and frostings.

Consuming too much trans fat raises your bad cholesterol level and increases your risk of heart disease. Try to limit trans fat intake to less than 1% of your daily calories. For someone on a 2,000-calorie diet, that's just 20 calories or 2 grams per day. It doesn't take much to reach that limit, so be attentive.

Here are a few practical tips:

- Limit fast food and highly processed snacks.
- Trim visible fats from meats.
- Read food labels carefully, especially for partially hydrogenated oils.
- Choose whole, natural foods whenever possible.

Keep in mind: if a food contains less than 0.5 grams of trans fat per serving, manufacturers aren't required to list it on the label. That means you could unknowingly exceed your daily limit just by eating common foods. So stay alert. Your choices matter.

Fats can either support or sabotage your health. Choose wisely. Choose strategically.

Water: The Overlooked Essential

Water is vital, not just for survival, but for overall wellness. Yet, it's often overlooked when discussing nutrition and weight management. Though it's not officially listed among the food groups, I believe water deserves a place on that chart. Its role in supporting the body's systems is just as critical as any nutrient found in food.

I have a strong personal preference for drinking plenty of water. I encourage you to do the same, especially between meals. This simple habit can help you feel full longer, reduce unnecessary snacking, and support healthy hydration. Choosing water over soda or sugary drinks is a powerful strategy for successful weight management.

To make this work, you'll need to be intentional. Start at a pace that feels comfortable for you. Over time, your body will adjust to regular water intake and begin to expect it.

Here's something important to understand: if you wait until you're very thirsty to drink water, your body is likely already dehydrated. Instead, take small sips throughout the day, even when you're not thirsty. This habit is especially important if you currently drink very little water.

When your water intake is consistently low, your body adapts by conserving what little it receives. Over time, your thirst cues may weaken, and your body will rely on minimal hydration, even though it needs more. This is a basic survival mechanism. The body will do its best with what it gets, whether it's nutrients or water. But this adaptation can lead to problems down the road.

The good news? You can retrain your body to accept and benefit from regular hydration. Of course, some individuals have medical conditions that require limited water intake. If your doctor has advised you to restrict fluids, follow that guidance. But if you're not in that group, drinking a reasonable amount of water daily will support your health.

For most adults, a good target is about eight 8-ounce glasses of water per day, roughly half a gallon or 2 liters. If you're exercising or spending time outdoors in hot weather, your body may need more. Pay attention to your body's signals. It will tell you what it needs. Listen!

You can even add water to your personal food group chart. It doesn't need to be a big production. It's on mine. When used wisely, water can benefit your body in countless ways. It supports digestion, metabolism, and energy levels. And yes, it can help you manage your weight and reach your wellness goals.

C – Consistency: Build Habits That Last

Now let's talk about the "C" in our ABCs, Consistency. This is where the magic happens. You can have all the knowledge and tools, but without consistency, results won't stick.

Consistency means showing up for yourself every day. It means making healthy choices most of the time, not all the time. It means building routines that support your goals. It's not about perfection, it's about persistence.

Let me re-share a personal example to support being consistent.

After I had my first child, I struggled with joint pain. I was breastfeeding and not getting enough calcium or vitamin D. I started taking a small supplement and adjusting my meals. I added leafy greens, dairy, and fortified foods. Slowly, the pain eased. My energy returned. And I felt strong again.

But it wasn't a one-time fix. It was a daily practice. I had to be consistent. I had to listen to my body and respond with care. I had to make small adjustments and stick with them. That's what I want for you; not a perfect plan, but a personal one. One that fits your life and evolves with you.

Consistency is also about being kind to yourself. Some days will be great. You'll eat well, hydrate, and feel amazing. Other days may be harder. You might skip a meal, overeat, or forget your water. That's okay. What matters is that you keep going. That you return to your habits quickly and keep building them.

Think of consistency as a rhythm. It's not rigid, it flows. It adapts. It grows with you. And over time, it becomes second nature.

Wrap-Up: Key Takeaways

- **You can eat and still lose weight.** Healthy eating is the most sustainable way to manage your weight.
- **Follow the ABCs of Nutrition:**
    - **(A) Awareness:** Understand what you eat and why. Pay attention to nutrients and how food affects your body.
    - **(B) Balance:** Include all food groups: fruits, vegetables, grains, protein, dairy, and healthy fats. Aim for appropriate portions. Avoid extremes.
    - **(C) Consistency:** Make healthy eating a lifestyle through habits that last.
- **Prioritize nutrition before calories.** Analyze the quality of your food first, then manage calorie intake for long-term success.
- **Fruits and vegetables are foundational.** Eat plenty, choose variety, and aim for whole forms for fiber and phytonutrients.
- **Choose smart carbs.** Focus on complex carbohydrates for sustained energy; limit refined sugars and processed foods.
- **Protein matters.** Include lean sources, legumes, and nuts. Watch portion sizes and aim for balance.
- **Dairy in moderation.** Opt for low-fat, low-sugar options and monitor calcium and vitamin D intake.
- **Healthy fats are essential.** Prioritize plant-based and fish oils; limit saturated and trans fats.

- **Water is non-negotiable.** Drink consistently to support hydration, digestion, and fullness.
- **Build your personal pyramid.** Keep YOU at the center of your nutrition plan for lasting success.

With these basics, you can confidently analyze any diet, meal, or trend. You'll make informed choices, build habits that last, and most importantly, achieve and maintain a Healthy Weight, without sacrificing your health.

You've now laid a strong foundation for healthy eating. You've connected nutrition to your goals and kept YOU at the center of the process. That's powerful progress.

Now, keep practicing awareness, balance, and consistency. These principles will help you create habits that support both weight and wellness. Remember, this journey isn't about perfection. It's about progress. Every choice you make moves you closer to your goals.

Stay focused, stay intentional, and keep moving forward. You've got this!

CHAPTER SIX

The Weight Management Trio

When you understand your hunger, honor your body, and add structure to your meals, real change happens. Satiety, Speed, and Snacking work together to keep you in control, not overwhelmed.

Plan your meals. This simple habit can help you avoid constant worry or preoccupation with food and your next meal. Being a planner supports both your health and your peace of mind. It's also important to create a structure; one that empowers you to make confident, healthy choices when faced with options. This chapter will help you build that structure successfully.

Let me start with a critical question, one that will challenge you to approach meals with deeper insight:

Why do you eat?

Yes, it's a simple question, but I imagine you have many answers. People eat for all kinds of reasons. Some eat out of boredom, others for comfort, and some simply because food is available. Now, here's a second question. Please answer this one with complete honesty:

Why do you think you *need* to eat?

Now let's talk a bit about hunger:

When it comes to hunger, this second question should take priority. Answering it helps you better understand your hunger cues and respond to them appropriately. Hunger is a powerful signal from your body, a cue that can drive you to eat in ways that may not serve your long-term wellness if misunderstood.

Eating is a basic human need. But sometimes, it's used to fill other unmet needs, especially emotional ones. This substitution can lead to problems, like eating when bored. Instead, meet boredom with fulfilling, self-building activities or hobbies.

Now, revisit your answer to that second question. Did you include these two reasons?

1. To satisfy hunger
2. To provide nutrients

These are the primary reasons we eat. Most people recognize #1, hunger, but often overlook #2, nutrients. Yet, meeting your body's nutritional needs is just as important. When your body gets the nutrients it needs, cravings for junk food decrease. You gain control and eat with intention.

With those two reasons in mind, let's explore three essential factors that will help you reach your weight loss goals. These factors also support the two key reasons you eat. I call them the Essential Trio of Weight Loss:

- Satiety
- Speed
- Snacking

Your success in managing your weight depends on understanding and managing this trio.

- Satiety refers to the feeling of complete satisfaction after eating.
- Speed is the rate at which your food digests; how long it takes before you feel hungry again.
- Snacking involves eating small amounts of food between regular meals.

Using these three strategically can help you make better food choices and stay on track with your goals. As we go further, I'll show you how to apply them practically.

Your major meals breakfast, lunch, and dinner, form the foundation of your daily intake. Snacks fill the gaps between these meals. By now, you should have a general idea of your daily calorie needs. Based on our earlier discussions, I'll use a reference range of 1,800–2,000 calories per day for an adult aiming for weight maintenance.

For weight loss, the approach is simple and practical: consume slightly fewer calories than your maintenance level daily. Do this gradually, cut back a little at breakfast, lunch, and dinner. I'll share strategies that help you reduce calories without stress. The goal is to build lasting habits that support your health.

Remember: the focus should be on YOU. Your strategies should revolve around your needs, not the other way around. Avoid drastic calorie cuts. They can deprive your body of essential nutrients and harm your long-term health. Your goal should be to reach your ideal weight while maintaining wellness. Never pursue weight loss at the expense of your health.

When planning your meals, fit your calorie targets into a nutrient-rich diet. I'll share what has worked for me over the years, explain why, and suggest ways you can tweak it to suit your lifestyle.

Wrap-Up: Key Takeaways

- **Understand why you eat.** Focus on hunger and nutrition as your primary reasons.
- **Use the Weight Management Trio.** Apply Satiety, Speed, and Snacking to guide your choices.
- **Plan meals and snacks with intention.** Support both health and weight goals.

Your next step is to apply these principles when planning your meals. This simple structure will help you stay in control and reduce stress around food decisions. Remember, progress comes from consistency, not perfection.

You're ready to move forward. Let's keep building habits that last!

Let's begin with breakfast.

CHAPTER SEVEN

Breakfast and YOU

How you start your morning shapes everything that comes after it. A breakfast built with intention, one that satisfies you, digests steadily, and reduces snacking, puts YOU back in charge of your day.

Breakfast is one of the most important meals of the day. It jumpstarts your metabolism after a long overnight fast, literally breaking your fast. When planning breakfast, keep the Essential Trio in mind:

- Satiety: Choose foods that help you feel full.
- Speed: Choose foods that digest gradually.
- Snacking: Choose foods that reduce the urge to snack before lunch.

Exploring the main food groups will help you make wise choices that support this trio. Choose whole grains, protein, and small amounts of healthy fats (monounsaturated and polyunsaturated). Whether it's cereal or pancakes, opt for whole grain components.

The 85:15 Rule

I teach a wellness concept called the 85:15 "Healthy vs. Unhealthy" Rule. Aim for at least 85% of your daily or weekly intake to come from healthy foods. The remaining 15% or less allows room for treats or indulgences. You can use this flexibility across meals, weekends, or spread it throughout the week. This approach gives you freedom, but also responsibility. It reminds you that YOU are in control, reducing stress and empowering better choices.

Another concept I teach is "being the boss of your body." You are the ultimate authority over what goes into your body. I explore this further in my book, *Healthy Me: Discovering Personal Health and Healing Naturally*. This mindset helps you use your 10–15% wisely and intentionally.

Sugar Awareness

Many of the people I've coached struggle with high sugar intake, especially at breakfast. It's one of the most common habits that quietly undermines weight loss goals. Why? Because added sugars can rapidly deplete your daily calorie quota without offering any meaningful nutrition. They fill you up with energy that burns fast and leaves you hungry again soon after.

We've already agreed that your focus should be on nutrition first, then calories. Trying to do it the other way around, counting calories without considering nutritional value, often leads to frustration and poor results. When you prioritize nutrition, you put YOU at the center of your choices. That's the first step toward sustainable weight and wellness management.

Let's talk about your taste buds. Did you know you can train your tongue to be satisfied with little or no sugar? Yes, and it's simpler than you might think. Start small. Try going a day or two without sweets. If that feels manageable, stretch it to a week. You'll be surprised how quickly your cravings begin to fade. Your taste buds will adjust, and foods that once seemed bland will start to taste naturally sweet.

When you return to your usual routine, take control of the sugar you add to your food. For example, if you enjoy cereal in the morning, try mixing unsweetened cereal with a small portion of sweetened cereal. Start with a 50/50 mix, then gradually increase the unsweetened portion. Choose whole grain varieties you enjoy, ones that support your digestion and help you feel full longer.

Whole grains are your ally. They promote gradual digestion, which is essential for effective weight management. Quick-digesting foods spike your blood sugar and leave you hungry again too soon. That's why it's important to cut back on syrups and other concentrated sugars at breakfast.

Also, be cautious with sugar substitutes. Not all are created equal. Avoid artificial sweeteners like aspartame and similar compounds, which may have negative effects on your health. Remember: your goal is wellness, not just weight loss. Don't sacrifice your health in the name of looking "cute" or chasing quick results.

Instead, explore natural alternatives. There are many healthier sweeteners available today. One option I often recommend is honey. It's very sweet, so a small amount goes a long way. Yes, it still contributes calories, but it also contains trace nutrients and is less processed than refined sugar. Use it sparingly and intentionally.

The key is to decrease sugar intake in ways that suit you. There's no one-size-fits-all approach. Explore your options, experiment with substitutions, and find what works best for your taste and lifestyle. Reducing sugar at breakfast is one of the most effective ways to lower your overall calorie intake, and it sets a positive tone for the rest of your day.

Protein at Breakfast

Protein should be a non-negotiable part of your breakfast. It's vital for health, and as we've discussed earlier, it plays a key role in digestion, satiety, and energy balance. Eating moderate amounts of protein in the morning helps your body digest food at a steady pace, keeping you full longer and reducing the urge to snack before lunch.

At any meal, aim for 10 to 25 grams of protein. For breakfast, a range of 10 to 17 grams is a solid start. Some days may vary, and that's okay. Try not to go below 10 grams. When combined with fiber from whole grains, fruits and vegetables, and healthy fats, protein helps slow digestion and stabilize your energy levels throughout the morning.

Meals that rely heavily on non-complex carbohydrates like white bread, sugary cereals, or pastries, digest quickly and leave you feeling hungry soon after. These foods lack the staying power that protein and healthy fats provide.

Milk is a great way to add protein and other nutrients to your breakfast. If you tolerate dairy, good-quality milk can be a valuable addition. Personally, I consume dairy in limited amounts to enjoy its benefits without overdoing it. As with most things in nutrition, moderation is key.

Building a Balanced Breakfast

On a typical busy weekday, I like to keep breakfast simple but intentional. I often reach for whole-grain cereal with milk, using about 80–90% unsweetened cereal and a small portion of sweetened cereal to control my sugar intake. When I can, I choose cereals with nuts for added protein and healthy fats.

Some days, I'm able to prepare eggs, which are a great source of protein. I also enjoy warm cereals like oatmeal or cream of wheat when time allows. These options are comforting, nutritious, and easy to customize.

Because I consume most of my dairy in the morning, I take a small dose of calcium (about 300 mg) with vitamin D at breakfast. This timing helps my body absorb the supplement more effectively, as it mimics the nutrients found in food. Some days, breakfast is the only time I consume dairy, so I use this opportunity to support my calcium needs.

On other days, I may include small amounts of cheese in snacks or later meals. However, those portions aren't always enough to meet my daily calcium requirements, which is why I supplement. When I take calcium with vitamin D, I do so alongside milk or dairy-containing foods to enhance absorption.

It's important to be strategic when taking supplements. The body absorbs nutrients best from food, so pairing supplements with meals can improve their effectiveness. Your doctor may advise you to take your multivitamin with food, depending on your health needs.

Here are a few key nutrient interactions to keep in mind:

- Calcium is best absorbed with vitamin D.
- Calcium competes with iron for absorption.
- Vitamin C enhances iron absorption.

I'll expand on these interactions in the lunch and dinner sections.

Whatever your breakfast looks like, aim to include:

- High-quality protein
- Complex carbohydrates
- Healthy fats
- Fruit (e.g., berries for fiber and antioxidants)

This combination will help you stay full longer, support digestion, and set a strong foundation for your day.

Water After Breakfast

Between breakfast and lunch, water becomes your best friend. Often, what feels like hunger is actually thirst. Drinking water first can restore the feeling of fullness and help you avoid unnecessary snacking.

Water also slows digestion, which supports the Essential Trio, especially Satiety and Speed. It's a simple yet powerful strategy for managing your weight and improving your overall health.

Here's something important to remember: your body adapts to what you give it. If you consistently drink small amounts of water, your body will adjust by conserving it. The kidneys will reduce urine output to preserve hydration. But this adaptation isn't ideal. It's a survival mechanism, not a wellness strategy.

Just because you're not thirsty doesn't mean your body doesn't need water. Water helps flush out toxins, supports cellular function, and keeps your systems running smoothly.

As we discussed earlier, aim for about eight 8-ounce glasses of water per day, roughly 2 liters or half a gallon. You don't need to drink large amounts all at once. Start with small, intentional sips and gradually increase the frequency. After breakfast, sip water regularly until lunchtime. Go at a pace that feels manageable.

This habit will help:

- Reduce snacking
- Support digestion
- Improve hydration
- Reinforce satiety

And here's a bonus tip: drink water when you snack, too. It enhances the effects of the Essential Trio and helps you stay in control of your hunger cues.

So, grab your water to go, right after breakfast. Use this to your advantage!

Breakfast Lounge Choices

Imagine walking into a breakfast lounge with limited time and several options in front of you. You need to make a quick decision, but one that supports your weight and wellness goals. Each option includes a small bowl of fresh fruit, and all portions are reasonably sized.

Here are your choices:

1. Donut and coffee with a fruit bowl
2. Whole grain pancakes with an egg, a glass of 2% milk, plus a fruit bowl
3. A bowl of whole-grain cereal (sweetened or unsweetened) with 2% milk, plus a fruit bowl

Discussion of Choices

Let's evaluate each option using the Essential Trio:

- Satiety – Will it keep you full?
- Speed – Will it digest gradually?
- Snacking – Will it reduce the urge to snack before lunch?

1. Donut and Coffee with a Fruit Bowl

At first glance, this option may seem satisfying. The fruit bowl and coffee can give you a quick feeling of fullness, so satiety is briefly addressed. However, this feeling won't last long. The donut is high in refined sugar and low in fiber, and it digests quickly. The fruit adds some fiber and nutrients, but the donut contributes mostly empty calories.

Most people add creamers to their coffee, which offer little nutritional value. Even if you add milk, it's usually a small amount, perhaps 2 ounces, which provides only 2 grams of protein. Compare that to a full glass of milk, which offers 8 grams.

The donut is also deep-fried, contributing unhealthy fats. These foods digest quickly and don't support long-term fullness. Without enough protein, fiber, or healthy fats, this meal fails the Speed test. Digestion will be rapid, and hunger will return soon.

And when hunger returns quickly, snacking becomes inevitable. So, this choice fails both the Speed and Snacking tests, passing only Satiety, and only temporarily.

Verdict: This is not an ideal choice for weight management. If you enjoy donuts and coffee, reserve this option for rare occasions. Repeatedly choosing this meal can lead to poor outcomes. Think nutrition first, then taste, and finally calories.

2. Whole Grain Pancakes with Egg, Milk, and Fruit Bowl

This option is nutrient-rich and well-balanced. The combination of solid food and liquid helps you feel full quickly, Satiety test passed.

The whole grain pancakes and fruit provide fiber, which supports digestion and fullness. The egg adds 6 grams of protein, and the glass of 2% milk adds another 8 grams, totaling 14 grams of protein. You also get a small amount of healthy dairy fat, which helps slow digestion.

This meal digests at a steady pace, keeping you full longer and reducing the likelihood of snacking, Speed and Snacking tests passed.

Verdict: This is an excellent choice, assuming clean ingredients in the pancake as well. It supports all three components of the Essential Trio and sets you up for a successful morning.

3. Whole-Grain Cereal (Sweetened or Unsweetened) with 2% Milk and Fruit Bowl

This option offers flexibility. Ideally, choose unsweetened whole-grain cereal, or mix a small portion of sweetened cereal with mostly unsweetened. This helps you reduce sugar intake while still enjoying the taste.

Cereals and beverages can be hidden sources of sugar, so always read labels. Choose cereals with natural ingredients, limited additives, and recognizable components. Think of your daily calorie quota as currency. Spend it on nutrients, not empty calories.

Unsweetened cereal helps you cut calories without sacrificing nutrition. You can train your taste buds to enjoy less sugar over time. The combination of cereal and milk provides solids and liquids, which support satiety, Satiety test passed.

Depending on the cereal, protein content can vary. Cereals with nuts or oats tend to have more protein, anywhere from 2g to 7g per serving. Let's assume your cereal has 5g of protein, and your milk adds 8g, totaling 13g of protein, comparable to the pancake and egg option.

This meal also contains fiber, dairy fat, and protein, which support gradual digestion, Speed test passed. With these components in place, the need for snacking is reduced, Snacking test passed.

Verdict: Another great choice. It's easy to prepare, customizable, and supports your weight and wellness goals.

These examples show that healthy breakfast choices are possible, even when you're short on time. Whether you prefer cereal or a warm breakfast, you can make smart selections that align with your goals.

Here's what to remember:

- Eat breakfast daily.
- Choose unsweetened cereals or mix them with sweetened ones.
- Look for cereals with protein, especially those with nuts or whole grains.
- Include fruit for fiber and nutrients.

Later, we'll explore lunch, dinner, and snacks, and how to use fruits strategically to support your wellness journey.

Morning Choices, Lifelong Impact

Take a moment to assess your current breakfast habits. Start by estimating your calorie intake. Read nutrition labels to get a clearer picture. Ask yourself:

- How much sugar do I consume at breakfast?
- Am I eating whole grains?
- Do I include protein and nuts?

Once you've answered these questions, look for ways to reduce added sugar. Try incorporating nuts and protein-rich foods, being mindful of any allergies. When available, choose options that include whole grains and fruits to boost your fiber intake. These choices will help you meet the Essential Trio criteria at breakfast:

- You'll feel full (Satiety).
- Your food will digest at a gradual pace (Speed).
- You'll be less likely to snack before lunch (Snacking).

Also, remember to drink water with purpose between breakfast and lunch. Sometimes, what feels like hunger is actually thirst. Staying hydrated supports digestion and helps regulate hunger cues.

If Your Goal Is Weight Loss

The strategies we've discussed can help you cut unnecessary calories and support gradual, sustainable weight loss. One effective approach is to reduce breakfast portions slowly. Many people struggle because they start with drastic cutbacks, which trigger strong hunger cues and lead to overeating later.

Instead, reduce portions in small increments. This gives your stomach time to adjust. Pair fiber-rich foods (like whole grains and fruits) with protein and healthy fats to increase satiety and slow digestion. These combinations help regulate hunger and support long-term weight management.

By following these strategies, you'll build lasting habits that not only help you reach a healthy weight but also enhance your overall wellness.

You can do this.

If Your Goal Is Weight Gain

If you're aiming to gain weight, the same principles apply. Just with a different focus. Start by ensuring your meals are nutritionally balanced. A well-rounded breakfast will help regulate hunger cues and support your energy needs.

Next, incorporate healthy, calorie-dense snacks throughout the day. Read labels carefully and choose options that align with your wellness goals. Estimate how many extra calories you need daily, and use those calories wisely, through snacks, healthy condiments, and nutrient-rich sides added to meals.

As you approach your goal, shift into maintenance mode. Your body will adapt to the changes you make, and you'll be able to sustain your progress with confidence.

Wrap-Up: Key Takeaways

- **Breakfast matters.** It jumpstarts your metabolism and sets the tone for your day.
- **Apply the Essential Trio:**
  - **Satiety:** Choose foods that keep you full.
  - **Speed:** Opt for foods that digest gradually.
  - **Snacking:** Reduce the urge to snack before lunch.
- **Follow the 85:15 Rule.** Aim for at least 85% healthy choices and allow 15% or less flexibility for treats.
- **Reduce added sugar.** Train your taste buds to enjoy less sweetness and choose natural alternatives like honey in moderation.
- **Prioritize protein.** Include 10–17 grams at breakfast to support satiety and energy balance.
- **Choose whole grains and healthy fats.** They slow digestion and help maintain fullness.
- **Drink water between meals.** Hydration supports digestion and reduces unnecessary snacking.
- **Make intentional choices.** Whether at home or on the go, select options that align with your wellness goals.

- **Adjust portions gradually.** For weight loss, reduce breakfast size slowly; for weight gain, add nutrient-rich snacks and sides.

Breakfast is your opportunity to fuel your body with intention. By focusing on satiety, speed, and smart choices, you'll build habits that support your weight and wellness goals. Remember, this isn't about perfection, it's about progress. Every small step counts.

Start tomorrow with a breakfast that reflects your goals. You've got this!

CHAPTER EIGHT

Lunch, Dinner, and YOU

Lunch and dinner give you the opportunity to build on the foundation breakfast set. With Satiety, Speed, and Snacking in mind, you create balance that supports you long after the meal is over.

You've made it to lunchtime, and you're not starving. That's a win! Your breakfast choices have set the tone, and now it's time to continue making smart decisions with YOU at the center. Just like breakfast, guide lunch and dinner with the Essential Trio:

- Satiety: Will it keep you full?
- Speed: Will it digest gradually?
- Snacking: Will it reduce the urge to snack between meals?

Use this trio as your compass, and you'll stay on track with your weight management goals.

Building Your Plate: The Four-Quarter Method

When preparing your lunch plate, visualize dividing it into four equal parts. This simple method helps you balance nutrients and stay aligned with your weight and wellness goals.

Quarter 1: Carbohydrates

Fill one quarter of your plate with complex carbohydrates and whole grains, as discussed earlier. These choices provide fiber, which supports all three components of the Essential Trio:

- Satiety: Helps you feel full
- Speed: Slows digestion
- Snacking: Reduces the urge to snack between meals

Whole grains also help stabilize blood sugar and provide sustained energy throughout the afternoon.

Quarter 2: Protein

The second quarter should include a good source of protein. Use our previous discussions as a guide and aim to limit highly processed proteins. I often say, *you can only do so much to process chicken and poultry compared to other meats.* That's why chicken and turkey are usually better choices.

If you're choosing beef, opt for slow-cooked preparations, especially if you didn't prepare it yourself. Cooking beef at high temperatures can produce harmful substances. I explore this further in my book, *Healthy Me: Discovering Personal Health & Healing Naturally*, where

I share tips on enjoying beef while minimizing potential exposure to these toxins.

If processed lunch meats are your only option, choose the least processed varieties. Be cautious. Most processed meats are low in protein per slice and high in sodium, which can quickly add up. Choose minimally processed deli meats when possible, and prioritize lean poultry.

If you must eat deep-fried chicken, remove the skin and coating. These tend to absorb lots of oil. Enjoy these foods occasionally, and limit deep-fried items overall. These small adjustments can help you cut unnecessary calories while still enjoying your meals.

Keep in mind: your protein intake at lunch plays a major role in satiety. If you had 10–17 grams of protein at breakfast, aim to get the bulk of your remaining daily protein from lunch and dinner. Pay attention to your protein intake. It matters.

Quarters 3 & 4: Fruits and Vegetables

The remaining half of your plate should be filled with fruits and vegetables. Fruits contain natural sugars which count toward your daily calorie limit, but they also come with valuable nutrients. Unlike processed sugary foods, fruits offer fiber, vitamins, and antioxidants that support your health.

That said, if your goal is weight loss, try to include more vegetables than fruit. Vegetables are typically lower in sugar and calories, while still offering a wide range of nutrients. Both fruits and vegetables belong to the same category on the food pyramid, so if only vegetables are available, that's perfectly fine.

Aim for variety. Different colors represent different nutrients, and a diverse plate supports overall wellness. Even if you take supplements, they should complement, not replace, good nutrition. Nutrients are best absorbed from food, especially when meals are well-balanced.

Some people eat well but don't combine foods in ways that enhance absorption. For example, vitamin C from fruits and vegetables helps your body absorb iron from protein and other sources. When you combine these foods thoughtfully, your body benefits more.

Moderate amounts of fruits and vegetables, paired with protein, will help you feel full after lunch or dinner. The fiber in these foods also supports digestion, helping food move steadily through your system. This contributes to both Satiety and Speed, and ultimately helps you pass the Snacking test as well.

The Power of Meal Complexity

Including a wide variety of fruits and vegetables in your meals increases the amount of fiber available to your body. This fiber plays a crucial role in helping you meet the Satiety test by keeping you full longer. It also supports the Speed test by promoting steady digestion. Fiber helps move food through the digestive tract in a smooth, consistent motion, which contributes to long-term digestive health.

Adding fruits and vegetables to your plate helps you pass both the Satiety and Speed tests. When these two are met, the need for frequent snacking naturally decreases. That means the Snacking test is also a pass. To support this process further, remember to drink water after lunch and dinner. Hydration helps reinforce satiety and supports digestion.

Fruits and vegetables are rich in vitamin C, which enhances the absorption of iron from your meals. Improved iron absorption can also support the uptake of other nutrients. Iron is essential for many bodily functions, including energy production and immune health.

From my coaching experience, I've found that digestion speed is one of the most important factors in successful weight management. A deeper understanding of this concept often marks a turning point for many people. That's why I emphasize both Speed and Satiety when discussing meal planning.

Timing matters. Each meal should include a balanced combination of protein and fiber, and when possible, small amounts of healthy fats. These components increase the complexity of your meal, which slows digestion and helps you feel full longer. You don't need to overcomplicate this. Just be mindful of choosing fats from healthy sources.

When meals contain sufficient protein, fiber, and healthy fats, digestion occurs at a steady pace. This helps prevent quick onset of hunger cues between meals, and reduces the likelihood of unnecessary snacking.

Some people eat carbohydrates alone, then add protein or fats later. However, carbohydrates digest much faster when consumed by themselves. This can lead to intense hunger shortly after eating and may result in frequent snacking or overeating. For those with specific lifestyle needs, eating six small meals a day may be more effective. Others do well with three main meals and small snacks in between. Whatever your routine, be intentional about making your meals and snacks nutritionally complex.

Include the components we've discussed: protein, fiber, and healthy fats, to build meals that support your goals. These choices will help you feel full, slow digestion, and maintain energy levels throughout the day. This is a key strategy for effective weight management.

Take a moment to reflect on your past habits. Can you identify any patterns or pitfalls? Now is a great time to create a plan that puts what you've learned into practice. Thoughtful meal planning and intentional choices will help you reach your weight loss goals more efficiently.

Using Fruits and Vegetables Strategically

Fruits and vegetables are powerful allies in your journey toward better health and effective weight management. Their vibrant colors are more than just visual appeal; they represent a variety of nutrients your body needs. Aim to include a wide range of colors in your meals, and always make room for your greens.

Enjoy both steamed and fresh vegetables, as each preparation method offers its own unique benefits. While I won't dive into the detailed nutritional breakdown here, it's important to keep in mind that variety matters. On most days, consider filling half of your plate with more vegetables than fruits. This approach provides excellent nutrition while limiting the natural sugars found in fruits, which can be especially helpful if your goal is weight loss.

That said, both fruits and vegetables offer valuable nutrients. Strive for balance. Be mindful of the natural sugars in fruit and how they contribute to your daily calorie intake. Some fruits contain more sugar than others, so it's helpful to account for their calories when planning your meals.

When preparing salads, pay attention to the dressings. Many store-bought options are high in calories and low in nutritional value. Look for smarter alternatives made with olive oil and herbs. You can even make your own at home using simple recipes from trusted cooking sites or books. Adjust them to suit your taste and your weight goals, using the tips you've learned throughout this chapter.

To further enhance your meals, consider adding plant-based proteins alongside your animal protein choices. Legumes such as beans, as well as nuts and seeds, are excellent sources of plant protein. Including these options not only boosts your protein intake but also adds variety and texture to your meals.

Smart Use of Fats and Oils

When planning your lunch and dinner, aim to include small to moderate amounts of healthy fats and oils. These are easy targets to meet, and as discussed earlier, healthy fats can play a significant role in supporting your wellness and making your weight goals more achievable.

Use the knowledge you've gained to guide your choices. Healthy fats can be incorporated throughout your plate in simple and effective ways. For example, you might use olive oil to sauté potatoes or stir-fry chicken. You can also add nuts and seeds to your salads, or include them in other parts of your meal. Avocado slices make a great topping and add both flavor and nutrition. Even your salad dressings can be a source of healthy fats when made with ingredients like olive oil and herbs.

Meeting both your calorie and nutrition goals is very doable when you pay attention to your selections. The key is to choose fats that offer nutritional value and to account for them in your daily intake. Think of your calorie quota as currency. Spend it wisely on foods that nourish your body, rather than on empty calories.

When selecting oils, choose the right kinds. A teaspoon of oil adds about 40 calories to your meal, while a tablespoon adds around 120. It doesn't take much to make a difference. Small amounts of healthy fats and oils can enhance your wellness without overwhelming your calorie budget.

Now imagine adding a tablespoon of olive oil to your lunch or dinner and pairing it with a sugary, empty-calorie drink. While this combination may significantly increase your calorie intake, it may still fall short of meeting your satiety needs if the meal lacks overall complexity. Healthy fats like olive oil can contribute to a satisfying meal, but they are most effective when combined with other essential components such as protein and fiber.

Without the right balance, digestion may occur too quickly, leaving you hungry again soon. This can lead to increased snacking or larger portions at your next meal, neither of which supports effective weight management. To avoid this, make sure your meals include elements that promote fullness. Protein, fiber, and healthy fats work together to slow digestion and help you feel satisfied for longer.

With thoughtful planning and smart choices, you can stay on track with your goals and build habits that support long-term wellness.

Watch Out for Add-ons

Be mindful of meal add-ons. These include condiments, salad dressings, drinks, and desserts. It's important to pay attention here, as I've found these to be common culprits that interfere with the weight management goals of many people.

Start by cutting back on some of these extras. You don't need to eliminate them all at once. Reduce them gradually and consider substituting with low-calorie, healthier alternatives. For example, try replacing sweetened drinks and sodas with water most of the time. Adding a few lemon slices can enhance the flavor of your water while also supporting your wellness goals.

If you choose to have sugary or less healthy beverages, limit each serving to about 2 to 3 ounces. One helpful strategy is to drink water first, which can reduce your desire for sweet drinks. The same applies to condiments. Many are high in calories and sodium, so cutting back can make a meaningful difference.

You can train your taste buds to align with your health goals. With time and intention, your preferences will shift. Use the knowledge you've gained to develop habits that support your wellness. Staying aware of these small choices will help you stay on track and maintain control over your weight goals.

Action Item: Making Smart Lunch & Dinner Choices

For most of us, lunchtime happens during the workday. You may have the option to pack your lunch or grab something from a nearby cafeteria or restaurant. The challenge with lunch is often time. Many people justify poor food choices because they're in a rush or trying to keep up with the demands of the day.

Just like with breakfast, it's important to stay aware of common lunchtime pitfalls. Whether you're packing your lunch or ordering takeout, choose foods that support your weight goals. The choices you make each day add up. As we've discussed, weight gain beyond your normal range often results from small, unhealthy decisions made consistently over time.

To lose weight, you need to reverse those patterns. Choose foods that promote weight loss and wellness. This approach will help you build habits that move you from your current state to your desired one, and help you maintain that progress once you get there.

Now, let's review a sample menu. You'll find options grouped into categories: meats, carbohydrates, fruits and vegetables, add-ons, drinks, and desserts. In real-life situations, these groupings may not be obvious. Use what you've learned to mentally sort items and make informed choices.

Sample Menu for Lunch or Dinner

Meats

- Grilled Chicken
- Baked Chicken
- Rotisserie Chicken
- Fried Chicken
- Chicken Wings
- Pot Roast
- Meat Loaf
- Steak
- Grilled Fish (various kinds)
- Fried Fish (various kinds)
- Baked Fish (various kinds)
- Beans (various kinds)
- Pork Chops
- Barbecue Ribs
- Sandwich Meats (processing level unknown)
- Burger Patties (processing level unknown)

Carbohydrates

- Potatoes (baked, mashed, sautéed with veggies)
- Sweet Potatoes
- Fries (sweet and regular)
- Chips (various kinds)
- Soft Tortillas (various kinds)
- Bread (whole grain and white)
- Pizzas (various kinds)
- Steamed Rice
- Steamed Corn

Vegetables and Fruits

- Fresh
- Steamed
- Canned
- Salad options

Add-ons

- Sour Cream
- Mayonnaise
- Pico de Gallo
- Salad Dressings (various kinds)
- Ketchup
- Cheese
- Mustard
- Dips (including veggie dips)
- Avocados
- Nuts (various kinds)
- Bacon Bits
- Ham
- Butter

Drinks

- Water
- Sodas (various kinds)
- 100% Fruit Juices (various kinds)
- Other Juices (various kinds)

Desserts

- Pastries (cakes, cookies, and other varieties)
- Ice Cream (various kinds)

Discussion & Personal Reflection

Have you made your choices? How does your lunch or dinner plate look? I imagine it's looking delicious. I've tried to include options that reflect what the average everyday plate might carry. If you've struggled with meal planning in the past, I hope this discussion has given you a few simple ways to start. From these ideas, you can explore recipes and adjust them to suit your weight management goals based on what we've covered.

Protein (Meat Choices)

As we've discussed, aim to eat healthy at least 85% of the time. This is based on my 85:15 "healthy versus unhealthy" concept. You can evaluate your choices weekly or daily, depending on your routine and preferences. The goal is to take control of what goes onto your plate at every meal. This ties into the concept of "being the boss of your body."

Start your lunch or dinner choices by reflecting on how much of your minimum of 85% healthy quota you've kept up with during the week. Most of the time, choose meats that are lean, minimally processed, and not deep-fried. This will naturally shift your preferences toward healthier options.

For chicken, try to limit deep-fried varieties to once or twice a week, or skip them altogether some weeks. The same goes for chicken wings. If that's your only option, remove the skin and dab off excess fat. Plan ahead for situations with limited choices, such as parties or events. Save your 10-15% indulgence quota for those occasions so you can enjoy them guilt-free.

With beef and similar meats, aim to limit consumption to one or two times per week. If you eat beef more often, choose slow-cooked options like pot roast, which are generally safer and better for your health. Select the least processed cuts, and when choosing burgers, go for pure meat patties. Limit charbroiled meats and steaks to just a few times per month, especially when dining out. If cooking at home, season with herbs like rosemary and thyme[1] to help reduce potentially harmful substances formed at high temperatures.

When it comes to sandwich meats, do your best to choose the least processed options most of the time.

For fish, prioritize baked, sautéed, or grilled preparations. These allow you to enjoy the benefits of fish oils without the added risks from deep-frying. If you eat fish regularly, aim for wild-caught varieties and limit farmed fish. Wild-caught fish generally contain fewer potential toxins. Remember, every food choice carries some level of risk and benefit. Your goal is to limit risks while boosting your body's ability to handle unavoidable exposures. Strengthen your immune system by making healthy choices at least 85% of the time.

At the grocery store, you can read labels and choose wild-caught fish. At restaurants, you may not know the source, but your other choices throughout the day or week can help you feel confident and guilt-free. What you eat most of the time matters. Be intentional with your choices, and your health will thank you. Take charge and be the boss of your body.

There are also various theories about eating scaled versus unscaled fish. Take time to read and explore these ideas, then make informed decisions about which types of fish to eat more often. Strive for the highest quality whenever possible.

In my book, *Healthy Me: Discovering Personal Health and Healing*, I explore wellness concepts such as Balance, Moderation, and Benefits versus Disadvantages. These ideas can help you navigate food-related dilemmas and make confident decisions. Learn more about these concepts to help answer your personal questions about meat and fish choices.

Are you satisfied with the meat choices on your plate? Do you need to make any changes based on what we've discussed? Make those adjustments before we move on to carbohydrates.

Carbohydrates

Let's take a closer look at your carbohydrate choices. For at least 85% of your lunches and dinners, aim for options that are whole and minimally processed. This aligns with our earlier discussion on carbohydrates and supports your weight and wellness goals.

Try to reduce your intake of deep-fried carbs. Planning ahead is key. A baked potato, for example, can be a great choice, but be mindful of the add-ons. These extras can introduce unhealthy ingredients, artificial additives, and empty calories. However, you can also use add-ons to your advantage. Fresh vegetables like Pico de Gallo can enhance flavor and nutrition. On the other hand, processed toppings such as bacon or ham are best limited or avoided.

If your plate is low in fats, a small amount of butter or cheese may be acceptable. The goal is to train your taste buds to align with your weight management goals. Start by cutting back on add-ons at one meal, then gradually reduce them over time. This includes salad dressings, which can be high in calories. Read labels when available and consider healthier substitutions. A few slices of avocado or a sprinkle of nuts and seeds can add healthy fats without overwhelming your plate.

Make these changes gradually. This gives your body time to adjust and helps you build habits that support long-term maintenance. Sweet potatoes are another excellent carbohydrate choice, offering great health benefits. Steamed corn is also a good option.

If you choose steamed rice, pair it with fiber-rich vegetables to help you feel full and avoid overeating. Most rice sold in stores is processed and low in fiber. To improve digestion and satiety, combine rice with beans, corn, or potatoes. You can also add steamed or sautéed vegetables to round out the meal. This strategy helps slow digestion and reduces your intake of refined foods.

Based on our discussion, do you feel ready to adjust your carbohydrate choices?

Fruits and Vegetables

You already know how valuable this section is to your weight goals. Fruits and vegetables help you pass the Satiety, Speed, and Snacking tests we've talked about. So, when it comes to this part of your plate, don't hold back, fill it up.

If you're choosing a tortilla, remember that it won't keep you full on its own. Add beans, vegetables, and even a bit of corn or rice from your carbohydrate portion to make the meal more complex and satisfying. Focus on building satiety through thoughtful combinations.

Watch out for add-ons that come with salads and vegetables, especially dips. These can add unnecessary calories. Instead, top your salads with a few nuts for healthy fats. You don't need many, just a small handful can make a difference.

Let your vegetable portions outweigh your fruit portions, especially if you're watching your sugar intake. Choose fresh produce whenever possible. If canned options are all you have, that's okay. Just balance it out in later meals.

Take a moment to reflect on your current choices. Do you need to make any changes or reconsiderations? Use the strategies you've learned to guide every plate you prepare. You'll be amazed at how far these small adjustments can take you in reaching your weight management goals. These are the habits that last a lifetime.

Add-ons, Drinks, and Desserts

Be mindful of add-ons. This can include condiments, salad dressings, drinks, and desserts. These are often overlooked but can significantly disrupt your progress with weight management. Another common challenge is snacking, which we'll discuss shortly. For now, keep it in mind as an area that deserves your attention.

Let's talk about desserts. Believe me, you don't need them with every meal. Most desserts offer little nutritional value and can easily be skipped without missing a thing. Ask yourself: why do you eat dessert? Is it to satisfy a sweet tooth? Or is it simply out of habit? I understand those moments and occasions when dessert feels appropriate, and yes, you can make room for it. But it doesn't need to be a daily routine.

Many people have developed the habit of eating dessert after lunch or dinner daily. Unfortunately, this can become an unnecessary addition to your daily calorie intake. The good news is that you can change this habit. It's not as difficult as it may seem. You've probably heard the phrase, "Out of sight, out of mind." If you don't buy or stock the foods you want to avoid, you're less likely to eat them. Start by limiting dessert to special occasions. You'll be surprised at how quickly your body and mind adjust.

Eventually, you'll find yourself naturally reducing your dessert intake, even when it's available. If your reason for dessert is to satisfy a sweet tooth, try cutting back gradually. Begin by reducing the portion size, then decrease how often you indulge. Desserts don't always have to be pastries. Consider healthier alternatives like sweet, seasonal fruits. A few pieces of fruit at the end of a meal can satisfy your cravings while supporting your wellness goals.

Personally, I reserve most desserts for gatherings with family and friends. I plan for them as part of my 10–15% "junk food" quota for the day, week, or month. Try this approach and see how your routine responds.

For example, if I plan to have dessert with lunch or dinner, I reduce or skip sugar in other meals that day. I also limit the portion and choose only the desserts I truly enjoy. The more "junk" you can train yourself not to crave, the better off you'll be. It starts with your mindset. Get intentional and begin to talk yourself out of the foods that no longer serve your goals.

After a satisfying lunch or dinner, grab a glass of water, just as you did after breakfast. This helps reawaken satiety between meals and keeps you feeling full longer. You'll notice less urgency to snack, if any at all. This strategy works well when practiced consistently.

The same principle applies to sugary drinks and alcohol. Alcohol contributes to your daily carbohydrate intake, and sugary drinks can add unnecessary calories. Even drinks labeled "100% juice" contain natural sugars. While these sugars have some nutritional value, they still count toward your daily limits.

Read labels carefully. Look for clean ingredients you recognize and understand. Some juices may offer 100% vitamin C, which is beneficial, but portion control is key. Limit juice consumption to small amounts, about 2 to 3 ounces per meal.

A helpful strategy is to always have water with your meals, regardless of what else you're drinking. Start by drinking more water. This will reduce cravings for juices and other sweet beverages and help you limit them to occasional sips. When you feel thirsty, reach for water first. Use this approach with any beverage you enjoy but know may not align with your health or weight goals.

If your goal is to gain weight, you may choose to drink milk or 100% juice when thirsty. If your goal is to lose weight or increase your water intake, try adding a few slices of lemon. Lemon offers great benefits for health and weight management and can be enjoyed by everyone who likes it. Squeeze some into your water when you can.

If you're working to reduce unhealthy drinks, include this in your weekly or monthly plan. Factor it into your 10–15% "junk" quota. You can schedule these drinks for special occasions or plan to enjoy them weekly, bi-weekly, or monthly, whatever suits your goals. Be intentional. Make a plan, stick to it, and remind yourself that you'll enjoy those drinks at your scheduled times. This will help you resist cravings in the moment.

Wrap-Up: Key Takeaways

- **Use the Essential Trio:** Plan lunch and dinner with **Satiety**, **Speed**, and **Snacking** in mind to stay full longer and reduce unnecessary snacking.
- **Apply the Four-Quarter Method:**
    - **Quarter 1:** Complex carbohydrates for fiber and sustained energy.
    - **Quarter 2:** Lean protein to support fullness and muscle health.
    - **Quarters 3 & 4:** Fill half your plate with fruits and vegetables for fiber, vitamins, and antioxidants.
- **Prioritize nutrient balance.** Combine protein, fiber, and healthy fats to slow digestion and maintain energy.

- **Choose healthy fats wisely.** Use small amounts of olive oil, nuts, seeds, or avocado to enhance nutrition without excess calories.
- **Watch add-ons and extras.** Condiments, dressings, sugary drinks, and desserts can add hidden calories. Reduce them gradually and choose healthier alternatives.
- **Practice the 85:15 Rule.** Aim for at least 85% healthy choices and allow 15% or less flexibility for treats.
- **Stay hydrated.** Drink water after meals and between meals to support digestion and satiety.
- **Plan for variety.** Include colorful fruits and vegetables, lean meats, and whole grains to maximize nutrient absorption and overall wellness.

Your lunch and dinner choices are powerful tools for weight management. By planning your plate with intention and practicing balance, you'll build habits that last. Remember, this isn't about perfection. It's about progress. Every smart choice moves you closer to your goals.

You can do this. Stay mindful. Apply these strategies, and you'll be well on your way to achieving your weight management goals.

CHAPTER NINE

Snacking and YOU

Smart snacking is a powerful tool. When you drink water first and choose foods that keep you full and focused when you need them, you turn snack time into a moment that works for you, not against you.

Snacking is a great topic to explore at this stage. It's the perfect time! When it comes to snacking, most of us fall into one of two categories:

- Habitual Snackers – Those who snack out of habit, often without hunger cues.
- Purposeful Snackers – Those who snack to sustain energy and bridge the gap to the next meal.

For effective weight management, the second category should be your goal. Which category do you fall into most often?

If you're in the first group, snacking out of boredom or just because food is visible, I want to raise your awareness.

I challenge you to move toward the second category. It's absolutely possible with intention. I've helped many people make this shift, and it makes a big difference in achieving weight goals. Start by making a decision now: become a purposeful snacker. In this chapter, you'll learn strategies to help you stay in control.

Start with Your Meals

Have you started applying what you've learned about breakfast, lunch, and dinner? If so, you're likely feeling satisfied and full after your meals. That fullness helps delay hunger cues between meals and supports sustained energy levels throughout the day. These benefits stem directly from the strategies we've already discussed.

However, if hunger strikes earlier than expected, you can still stay aligned with your weight management goals. Picture this: you are hungry, it's been a few hours since breakfast, but lunchtime is still a while away. What should you do first?

You guessed it; reach for your water and take a drink. This simple action can help "reawaken" your sense of fullness and may be all you need to feel satisfied again.

Water First, Always

After drinking water, you'll be better able to determine whether you truly need a snack. Often, what feels like the early signs of hunger is actually your body signaling a need for hydration.

For effective weight management, try not to rely on beverages other than water. Make it a habit to drink water first, even if you plan to have something like juice later. Starting with water can reduce how much of the other beverage you end up consuming. If your goal is to gain weight, you can reverse this approach.

This simple step can make a significant difference in your weight management plan. Drinking water between meals helps extend the time before your next hunger cue appears. It also slows the digestion of food still in your stomach, which supports the trio of satiety, speed, and snacking.

When You Truly Need a Snack

Let's say you've had water a third time after breakfast, and now you genuinely feel hungry. What should you do next? Would you reach for a bag of chips and a soda from the break room? That wouldn't be the best choice.

Also, remember to take a few sips of water before your main meals. This simple habit can help prevent overeating.

When it comes to snacking, keep Satiety and Speed in mind. These two are closely connected to smart snacking. Choose snacks that help you feel full and digest slowly. Think about protein, fiber, and healthy fats, just as we've discussed earlier.

What snacks come to mind when you focus on these three? You might consider:

- Nuts (whole or in butter form)
- Dairy options like cheese and milk
- Small portions of lean meats when available
- Fresh vegetables with healthy dips
- Fruits

As you make your choices, keep variety, moderation, and balance in mind. Reading labels can help you stay within your calorie goals and make informed decisions.

And don't forget, drink water after your snack. This will support satiety and help slow digestion, reinforcing your weight management strategy.

Planning for Treats

There will be days when you crave chips, and that's perfectly okay, as long as you plan with intention. When choosing chips, opt for whole-grain and baked varieties most of the time. If you decide to include less nutritious options, make sure they fit within your 10–15% treat quota.

Keep in mind that growing children and teens can handle occasional junk food more easily than adults. Moderation is key.

Even on days when chips are part of your plan, consider pairing them with vegetables or fruits. You'll likely find that you eat fewer chips when they're accompanied by more nutrient-dense foods.

If you have a large bag of chips, portion out the amount you intend to eat and then put the bag away. If you must eat directly from the bag, stay mindful of how much you're consuming and avoid going overboard.

Snack Frequency and Portion Control

When it comes to snacking, it's important to pay attention to both how often you snack and how much you eat. One effective way to reduce unnecessary snacking is by making smart choices during your main meals. As we've discussed, breakfast, lunch, and dinner should leave you feeling satisfied. When meals are well-balanced, you're less likely to feel hungry between them.

Keep in mind that snacks are not meant to replace meals. Their purpose is to lightly line your stomach and help you stay energized until your next meal. If you rely on snacks to fill you up like a meal, you may end up consuming more calories without feeling truly full.

To avoid overeating, take a moment to plan your snack or meal before you begin eating. Identify all the components ahead of time. This simple strategy increases awareness and helps you stay in control, especially on days when you're tempted to go back for seconds.

Be sure to include snack calories in your daily totals and track them. If mealtime is approaching, consider skipping the snack and having your meal a little earlier. When a snack is needed, choose foods that support your energy and focus.

A Real-Life Scenario

You're at work, and it's been about 3.5 hours since lunch. You notice a slight feeling of hunger, though you're not entirely sure. Drawing from what you've learned, you reach for a bottle of water and take a few sips. After drinking, you realize that you are indeed hungry and could use a snack. Dinner is still about 3.5 hours away.

You head to the break room and discover that someone has ordered snacks for the entire team. Here are the available options:

- Beverages: sodas, juices, coffee, and various teas
- Fresh fruits: apples, oranges, strawberries, pineapples, grapes, blueberries
- Veggie tray:
- Assorted vegetables such as broccoli, carrots, celery
- Dips including guacamole, queso, cheese, and others
- Chips: whole-grain, baked, and regular potato chips
- Crackers and cookies: assorted varieties
- Peanut butter
- Cheese slices
- Yogurt: various types
- Nuts: assorted kinds

What do you choose? Would you keep the concepts of Satiety and Speed in mind? If so, are you thinking about protein, fiber, and healthy fats? Excellent thinking.

Let's walk through a brief analysis to support your choices. Snack time tends to be quick, and since you've already mastered the principles around breakfast and lunch, selecting snacks should feel much easier.

Start with a beverage. Water is always a reliable choice. If you have room for something extra, apply what you've learned about beverages to stay aligned with your weight management goals. Drinking water before reaching for snacks is a smart first step.

Next, consider protein. This might lead you to options like peanut butter, cheese, or yogurt. These can be great choices, depending on your preferences and what you've already eaten today or earlier in the week.

Know your daily calorie limits and your ideal intake quotas. When choosing snacks, aim for options that leave room for dinner. You only need small portions, so avoid going overboard. Read labels carefully and watch for added sugars, especially in flavored yogurts. A smarter option would be plain yogurt with fresh fruit added. This allows you to use your calories in a way that supports both health and weight goals.

For fiber, include vegetables, fruits, or a few whole-grain crackers or baked chips. These choices help you feel full and support digestion.

When it comes to healthy fats, grab a small handful of nuts you enjoy. Even five nuts can make a difference. Small amounts go a long way. You might also add a teaspoon of guacamole to your veggies for an extra boost. Keep in mind that dairy options like yogurt or cheese also contribute to your fat intake. Watch out though, some types of dairy may contain unhealthy fats, so choose carefully.

If you have room within your 10–15% treat quota, you can consider regular chips, crackers, or cookies. These can occasionally replace whole-grain options. Just be mindful of portion sizes. Snack calories can add up quickly, so pay attention. If you want to sample a variety of snacks, substitute smaller portions to stay within your goals.

This is snacking simplified. If your goal is to gain weight, you can add extra calories from snacks.

You're all set. Grab a little more water as you leave the break room. The choices you've made will support satiety and digestion until dinner.

Now, let's pause for a moment. On most days, snack time won't offer such a wide variety of options. This scenario is special, but it does happen from time to time. What's common to all snack times is their brevity. Quick decisions don't lessen their value. In fact, brief moments like these are opportunities to practice smart habits.

Use this scenario to prepare for those everyday snack moments. Make choices that are quick, intentional, and supportive of your goals. For example, if you're thinking about crackers, reduce the number and top them with cheese or peanut butter. Add a few carrots, and keep your water close.

How does that sound? Quick, simple, and smart. That's what your snack times should look like. You can do this. You have what it takes.

Wrap-Up: Key Takeaways

- **Shift from habitual to purposeful snacking.** Snack to sustain energy and bridge the gap between meals, not out of boredom or habit.
- **Start with water.** Drink water first when hunger strikes; often thirst is mistaken for hunger.
- **Apply the Essential Trio:**
    - **Satiety:** Choose snacks that keep you full.
    - **Speed:** Opt for foods that digest gradually.
    - **Snacking:** Use snacks strategically to avoid overeating.
- **Focus on nutrient-rich snacks.** Include protein, fiber, healthy fats such as from nuts, yogurt, cheese, lean meats, fruits, and vegetables.

- **Plan for treats.** Use your 10–15% quota for indulgences like chips or cookies, and pair them with healthier options.
- **Practice portion control.** Avoid eating directly from large packages; measure out what you need.
- **Track snack calories.** Include them in your daily totals and adjust as needed.
- **Stay hydrated.** Drink water after snacks to enhance satiety and slow digestion.
- **Make quick, intentional choices.** Even brief snack moments can support your goals when approached mindfully.

Most snack times aren't as elaborate as the scenario we discussed, but the principles remain the same: quick, smart decisions. For example, if you want crackers, cut back on the number and top them with cheese or peanut butter. Add a few carrots and keep water nearby.

That's what smart snacking looks like; brief, intentional, and satisfying.

Smart snacking is about planning and awareness, not perfection. Every time you choose water first, pair treats with healthier options, and keep portions in check, you strengthen habits that last.

Stay intentional, stay consistent, and keep moving toward your goals. You've got this!

CHAPTER TEN

Weight and Habits: The 85:15 Concept

What you do most of the time determines where your health goes over time. The 85:15 concept helps you see your patterns clearly and shift them with intention.

Your actions and choices play a powerful role in shaping your habits. Over time, they can influence your life in either a helpful or harmful way. Interestingly, habits often begin to influence your choices even more than the other way around. Choices and habits feed off each other, forming patterns that can significantly impact your health.

Many people experience fluctuations in weight because they overlook what they do most of the time. The clue here is MOST TIMES. The 85:15 concept will help you visualize how this pattern shows up in everyday life and guide you toward more consistent, health-supporting habits.

Reflect on Your Daily Patterns

Let's begin with a simple but important exercise. Take a moment to reflect on the choices you make regularly regarding your health. Consider what you eat most of the time, your activity level, and how you manage stress. Journal the major patterns you notice in these three areas. Feel free to add more as they come to mind, especially as you begin to understand why this step is so important for maintaining a healthy weight.

Once you've written them down, ask yourself: How have these choices affected my health and weight?

Understanding the 85:15 Concept

Now that you've identified your patterns, let's explore how the 85:15 concept applies to them. This principle helps you evaluate your habits and understand their impact on your weight management goals.

You may recall the minimum 85:15 "healthy vs. unhealthy" rule from earlier chapters. It's a helpful guide for making food choices, but it can also be applied to other areas of life that influence your health habits.

The goal is to lean toward the healthy side, aiming for at least 85% of your choices to support your health. What you do most times matters, and this ratio helps you stay on track.

Applying the Concept to Positive Habits

Let's look at physical activity as an example of a positive habit. Regular movement supports your health and can be measured using the 85:15 guideline.

Try to get 30 to 60 minutes of aerobic exercise each day, aiming for 3 to 5 days per week. Your weekly goal should be around 150 minutes of moderate activity. If your workouts are more intense, 75 minutes per week may be enough. A mix of both is ideal, as long as it's safe and manageable for you.

Using a 7-day week as a reference, 85% of 7 days equals approximately 5.95 days. Even 75% comes to about 5.25 days, close to 5 days. This assumes 30 minutes of daily exercise. If your workouts are longer or more intense, fewer days may be needed. Either way, this meets the "most times" guideline and supports your health goals.

You can apply this concept to many areas of your life to strengthen your health habits.

Managing Negative Habits

Let's now take a closer look at a common negative habit: worrying thoughts. This ties directly into how you manage stress and can significantly affect your overall well-being.

Start by identifying a situation that has bothered you recently. How often do you find yourself thinking about it? Estimate how many minutes per hour you spend worrying, not problem-solving, just dwelling on the concern.

If you notice that you're spending 30 minutes of every hour worrying, it's time to reduce that to just 5 minutes. Unlike physical activity, worry does not support your health. To shift toward a healthier pattern, you'll need to actively cut back on the time spent in worry.

For habits like this, the goal is to reduce the time and replace it with healthier, more constructive thoughts. Even 15 minutes of worry per hour takes up a quarter of your time. In terms of the 85:15 concept, that would be a 75:15 ratio within a single hour. That is already too much. These minutes can quickly accumulate throughout your day.

Use your waking hours as a reference point to assess the impact of these habits. Seeing the numbers laid out can be a powerful motivator to take action.

Begin replacing worry with positive, solution-focused thoughts. This shift will help you move toward the healthier side of the 85:15 balance and support your overall weight and wellness goals.

Put the Concept into Practice

Now that you've explored both positive and negative habits, it's time to apply the 85:15 concept to your own life.

Return to your notes from the earlier reflection. Review the habits you recorded; those related to food, activity, stress, and any other patterns you identified.

Apply the 85:15 concept to each one. Keep practicing until it becomes second nature to evaluate your choices through this lens.

Hints:

- Positive Habits: These are the habits you want to strengthen. They include nutritious food choices and regular physical activity. Use the examples provided to guide your review.
- Negative Habits: These are the habits you want to reduce or manage more effectively. Stress-related habits, like worry, fall into this category. Use the stress example to help you reflect and adjust.

Wrap-Up: Key Takeaways

- **Your choices shape your habits.** What you do most of the time matters for your health and weight goals.
- **Apply the 85:15 rule.** Aim for at least 85% of your choices to support health, leaving 15% or less for flexibility.
- **Reflect on your patterns.** Identify habits related to food, activity, and stress, and assess their impact on your wellness.
- **Strengthen positive habits.** Include nutritious meals and regular physical activity. Aim for at least 150 minutes of moderate intensity exercises weekly.
- **Reduce negative habits.** Cut back on stress-driven behaviors like excessive worry and replace them with constructive thoughts.
- **Use numbers as motivation.** Seeing how much time unhealthy habits consume can inspire change.
- **Practice consistently.** Apply the 85:15 concept daily until it becomes second nature.

Your habits are powerful. They can work for you or against you. By leaning toward healthy choices most of the time, you'll create a lifestyle that supports your weight and overall well-being. Remember, this isn't about perfection; it's about progress.

Start today by reviewing your patterns and applying the 85:15 principle where it matters most. Every intentional choice brings you closer to your goals. You've got this!

CHAPTER ELEVEN

Influencers of Good Eating Habits

The more you understand what drives your hunger and cravings, the more control you gain over your eating habits. Knowledge turns confusion into clarity and puts YOU back in charge of your wellness journey.

There are several key factors that play a significant role in weight management. Understanding these influencers can empower you to make better choices and take control of your wellness journey.

Among the most important are hormones that regulate appetite and cravings. When you understand how they work, you can use that knowledge to your advantage.

Let's revisit a foundational concept from our earlier discussions: protein is essential for hormone production.

When you consume protein, your body breaks it down into amino acids. These amino acids are used to build various structures, including components that support critical functions. There are many types of amino acids, and eating a variety of protein sources helps ensure your body receives what it needs.

One of protein's key roles is supporting the formation of hormones. Eating clean, balanced meals gives your body the tools it needs to function well and sustain your energy. What you've learned so far is a valuable foundation for your long-term wellness goals.

Understanding Ghrelin and Leptin

Two important hormones help regulate your appetite[1]: ghrelin and leptin. These hormones work in opposite ways to manage hunger and fullness, using complex signals throughout the body.

Ghrelin is often referred to as the "I am hungry" hormone. It plays several roles, but its primary function is to stimulate appetite. It increases food intake and promotes fat storage. The stomach is the main producer of ghrelin, although small amounts are also released by the small intestine, pancreas, and brain.

Ghrelin triggers hunger pangs and signals the body to release stomach acids in preparation for digestion. If food is present, digestion begins. If not, those acids can irritate the stomach lining, leading to discomfort that compels you to eat.

This connects directly to our earlier discussion on satiety, speed, and snacking. Foods that slow digestion such as fiber from fruits and vegetables, along with protein and healthy fats, help you feel full for longer. They give stomach acids something to work on, which reduces cravings and the urge to snack. These three concepts are essential tools for supporting your weight goals.

It's also important to understand that hunger pangs don't always mean your body truly needs food. Other factors can trigger these sensations, including dehydration, lack of sleep, and even the smell of food[2]. Eating refined carbohydrates on their own can also lead to a quicker return of hunger.

As a word of caution, avoid responding to hunger pangs too quickly. If you do not have diabetes or other health concerns, take a moment to assess your situation. Drink water first and consider when you last ate. Hunger is not an emergency, and you can choose to wait if eating isn't necessary.

Remember your smart snack strategies. They are a top priority. Use them to your advantage.

Smart Pairing and Blood Sugar Control

Some foods cause a rapid spike in blood sugar followed by a sharp drop, which can lead to increased hunger. This is especially true for foods that are low in fiber, low in protein, or highly processed. These types of foods often result in excessive eating because they don't keep you full for long.

Take juice, for example. Drinking juice alone as a snack won't sustain you. Some people juice fruits and vegetables to support their health, especially in the morning or during specific wellness routines. Those who do this regularly are usually aware that juices digest quickly. Whether the juice is natural or not, you'll likely feel hungry again soon after drinking it.

That's why it's best not to rely on juice alone when you're hungry. Instead, pair it with fiber and protein to help you feel satisfied longer. A more effective approach is to enjoy juice alongside a balanced meal that includes protein and complex carbohydrates. This is especially important if you're working on managing your weight.

To clarify, this advice doesn't apply to occasional juice for pleasure or to structured juicing routines aimed at boosting health. It applies when you're feeling hungry and considering juice as a snack, even though other options are available.

Even natural juice contains calories, and depending on the type, those calories can be high. When juice is paired with a complex meal or snack, and especially if you drink water first, you'll likely consume less. This helps you stay within your calorie goals and make the most of your nutritional choices.

Use your calorie quotas wisely. Smart pairing makes a meaningful difference.

Leptin: The "I Am Full" Hormone

Leptin works in contrast to ghrelin and is often referred to as the "I am full" hormone. It acts as an anti-hunger signal. Leptin is produced primarily by fat cells in adipose tissue throughout the body. Its role is to signal the brain that the body has sufficient energy stored, reducing the need to consume more food.

Research on obesity has focused heavily on both ghrelin and leptin. Many studies have linked these hormones to habits that contribute to weight gain. In some cases, researchers have identified a condition known as leptin resistance, which has been associated with obesity[3]. This is similar to the concept of insulin resistance seen in some individuals with diabetes.

I use this comparison intentionally to highlight how your habits can directly influence your weight goals. Lifestyle choices play a significant role in hormone function. Poor habits can lead to leptin resistance, making it harder for the body to recognize fullness and regulate appetite effectively.

Your food choices matter. Following the guidance we've discussed will help you build positive, long-term habits that support your health and weight management goals.

Building Habits That Last

The most effective way to manage your weight is by building habits that are both positive and lasting. While some people undergo bariatric surgery or follow extreme weight loss programs, many eventually regain the weight they lost. These approaches can produce dramatic results, but without strong, supportive habits in place, those results are difficult to maintain.

Sustainable weight management requires empowering habits that support long-term success. Without them, even the most drastic changes tend to fade over time.

What you've learned throughout this book will help you lose weight and maintain it in healthy, realistic ways.

These strategies are designed to support lasting change and help you build a lifestyle that works for you.

Cravings and Brain Hormones

Brain hormones such as dopamine and serotonin play a key role in food cravings. The areas of the brain responsible for pleasure, memory, and reward also influence what and when you crave certain foods. It's important to understand that cravings are not the same as hunger pangs. Do not confuse the two.

Food cravings stem from these brain chemicals and create a strong desire for specific foods. This is a mental urge to satisfy a want, not a physical need. Cravings for items like chips, cookies, and cakes are often driven by dopamine and serotonin, which seek to fulfill brain-stimulated pleasures. The more you feed these cravings, the stronger they become.

The next time you experience a craving, remember that it is fueled by hormonal activity. Simply being aware of this can help you take control. Your goal is to build habits that rise above these urges. Use the concept of being the "boss of your body"[4] to help you stay empowered and intentional.

Continue practicing the principles of satiety, speed, and snacking. These three tools are essential and will give you an advantage in managing your weight and responding to cravings. Be mindful of your choices. Hormonal imbalances, including those involving leptin, can also contribute to cravings. Awareness is the first step toward change.

The Power of Smart Eating

One of the most encouraging truths about weight management is that smart eating can help you respond more effectively to hunger cues. It also plays a key role in balancing hormones. These two benefits work together in a cycle. Each one reinforces the other.

When you eat junk food, your body tends to crave more of it. On the other hand, when you choose healthy foods, your cravings for junk begin to fade. This is why balance is so important.

You don't need to understand every detail of how hormones drive cravings. What matters most is mastering the foundational concepts we've discussed, especially choosing the right foods for your plate. With frequent and intentional practice, you can develop this skill. And with consistent effort, you'll begin to see meaningful results.

Wrap-Up: Key Takeaways

- **Hormones influence appetite and cravings.** Ghrelin signals hunger, while leptin signals fullness; understanding these help you make smarter choices.
- **Protein matters.** It supports hormone production and overall wellness, so include a variety of protein sources in your meals.
- **Apply satiety, speed, and snacking.** Choose foods that slow digestion and keep you full longer to reduce cravings and unnecessary snacking.
- **Drink water first.** Hydration can curb false hunger cues and support digestion.

- **Pair foods wisely.** Combine fiber, protein, healthy fats and complex carbs to stabilize blood sugar and maintain fullness.
- **Watch out for quick-digesting foods.** Juices and refined carbs can spike blood sugar and lead to hunger soon after.
- **Leptin resistance is real.** Poor habits can disrupt fullness signals; healthy choices help restore balance.
- **Build habits that last.** Extreme diets or surgeries fail without strong, sustainable habits.
- **Cravings are hormonal, not hunger.** Dopamine and serotonin can drive cravings; awareness helps you take control.
- **Smart eating creates a positive cycle.** Healthy choices reduce junk cravings and support hormonal balance.

Your food choices are powerful tools for managing hunger, cravings, and overall health. By practicing smart eating and building habits that last, you'll create a lifestyle that supports your weight and wellness goals.

Start today; choose balance, hydration, and nutrient-rich meals. Every intentional choice brings you closer to success. You've got this!

CHAPTER TWELVE

Your Food Preferences

You're not powerless against your cravings or dislikes; you've been shaping your food choices since childhood. Now it's time to use that same power to choose what supports your health, not just what satisfies your habits.

Food Preferences Begin Early

How often do you hear someone say, "I don't like this," during a meal? Most people divide foods into two categories: likes and dislikes. This habit begins early in life. Toddlers often experiment with food preferences as part of their development. It's their way of managing the overwhelming choices around them and exercising control over their environment. When presented with food options, toddlers use these decisions to practice independence. Eating is a basic need, so it's natural for them to assert control in this area more than others. As they grow, reasoning skills improve, and they learn to apply control in other parts of life.

Control Over Food Choices Persists

Even as adults, a part of us still seeks to protect that sense of control over food, often without realizing it. Many toddlers reject foods without even trying them. Over time, some discover what they've been missing, but others never give certain foods a chance. This pattern can persist into adulthood. When the foods being rejected are unhealthy, that's not a problem. In fact, go ahead and dislike candies and cakes! The more you add to your "dislike" list of sweets, the better. This can work in your favor. Use this natural ability to shape your food choices for wellness and weight management.

Train Your Mind for Better Choices

You can train your mind to avoid foods that do not support your health goals. Deep down, you have the ability to control what enters your body. Some people have a stronger sense of control, but you can develop yours with practice. Start small, one plate at a time, one meal at a time, one decision at a time. This is doable, and you can succeed.

Reverse the Pattern

Eating only what you enjoy often leads to overeating. You can discipline yourself to eat what is good for you, even when it's not your favorite. Use your natural ability to control food choices in reverse: choose what you normally avoid when it benefits your health. Over time, this reverse technique becomes easier. It starts with mindfulness.

You are in control. You can give your body what it needs. Practice the concept of *being boss of your body*. Aim for 80–90% of your meal plan to include both your favorite and non-favorite healthy foods. This balance will help you stay on track with your weight management goals.

Portion Sizing and Long-Term Benefits

Portion sizing offers long-term benefits with weight management. Start by defining your normal plate size, based on earlier discussions. Your stomach will adapt to normal meal sizes if you avoid large portions consistently. This adjustment matters even when you eat foods you love. Over time, you'll train your stomach to feel content with reasonable portions. Even on days when you enjoy your favorites, smaller portions will satisfy you. Your stomach will signal "I'm full" at the right time. When you get that cue, respect it, especially when your plate is filled with favorites.

Wrap-Up: Key Takeaways

- **Food preferences start early.** Childhood habits often shape adult eating patterns.
- **Control over food choices persists.** Use this natural tendency to favor healthy options and limit unhealthy ones.
- **Train your mind for better choices.** Practice mindful eating, one plate, one meal, one decision at a time.
- **Reverse the pattern.** Don't eat only what you like; include healthy foods you normally avoid to support your goals.

- **Aim for balance.** Strive for 80–90% of your meals to include both favorite and non-favorite *healthy* foods.
- **Respect fullness cues.** Smaller portions and mindful eating help train your stomach for long-term success.

You have the power to shape your eating habits. By practicing mindfulness and making intentional choices, you'll create a lifestyle that supports your health and weight goals. Start small, stay consistent, and remember, you're the boss of your body.

You've got this!

CHAPTER THIRTEEN

Weight and Feelings

Your emotions and your weight are connected. When you learn to guide your feelings with intention, you strengthen the habits that move you closer to the healthy, confident version of YOU.

Feelings Matter in Weight Management

If your goal is a healthy weight, don't overlook your emotions. They play a bigger role than you might think. Positive feelings often go hand in hand with better health and wellness. When you align your emotions with your weight goals, you set yourself up for long-term success. Weight management is not just about food and exercise; it requires a holistic approach, and your emotional health is a vital part of that journey.

Your Unique Value

Always remember that you are unique. There is no one else on this planet exactly like you. If you ever doubt this, just look at your thumbprint. Did you know that someone can identify and separate you from the entire world population using your DNA-related data? Your unique identifiers confirm your individuality. You are valuable and have a unique potential to contribute to this world. There are things only you can do. Position yourself to be the best version of you.

How you feel about yourself is crucial. Your self-perception affects your ability to do everything you need to function. Sometimes, feelings can interfere with weight management. For many people, an obsession with weight management becomes a problem, especially when they lack a healthy approach. There is a right way to do everything, and there is a healthy way to manage your weight. This healthy approach truly works. It is the best way to take charge of your weight effectively. How you feel about yourself matters.

Emotional Health and BMI

Your emotional health plays a significant role in your ability to stay within the recommended BMI range of 18.5–24.9. Maybe you've calculated your BMI and found that you are outside this range. Don't worry about that. You have already made the right choice by deciding to reach your goal. Taking the first step is what matters. You won't stay where you are. That's why you are reading this book; to find strategies that will help you achieve your goals.

Planning and Progress

Worrying does not change anything. Instead, focus on planning well. Planning is the first step toward making real changes. Once you have a plan, you can let go of worry and concentrate on taking small steps, one at a time. Each step brings you closer to your destination.

Stay focused. That is all you need. Look ahead and keep your attention on the future. There is no benefit in worrying about the past, since you cannot go back and undo it. Put your energy into what lies ahead. You have the power to shape your future through the small steps you choose to take.

Use the practical strategies discussed in this book. From what you've learned, you can develop lifelong habits that will support you in the long term. You can reach your weight goals and maintain a healthy weight that helps you feel great in your body.

Reflecting on Your Number and Feelings

Now that you have your calculated number, pause and consider how you feel about it. Where do your feelings fit among these options: Great, Good, Indifferent, or Bad? Everyone finds themselves somewhere on this scale.

Once you identify your feeling, make it your goal to move away from "Bad" and toward "Great." Where you start is not as important as where you are headed. Our goal is to arrive at "Great."

For most people, feelings tend to align with their weight goals. Your feelings have a significant impact on your overall wellness. Be mindful and manage your emotions so you feel good most of the time. Awareness of your feelings will help you enjoy the journey of managing your weight and allow you to reach your goals with joy.

Feelings, Hormones, and Health

Try not to obsess over your calculated numbers. Your feelings influence your emotions, and this can affect your hormones and overall health. Hormones work together in the body, depending on each other and never acting in isolation. When hormones interact, they feed off each other, which determines the output of each hormone. Sometimes, the body produces certain hormones based on the levels of others, responding to signals to make more or less as needed.

Specific actions in the body can stimulate the production of particular hormones. In turn, some hormones can stop or encourage other actions. For example, consider the hormones ghrelin and leptin, which were discussed earlier. They operate in a loop, much like your thoughts, feelings, and emotions. These three also feed off each other, interacting at the cellular level and working together in cycles.

A positive thought can boost serotonin, known as the "feel-good hormone." This has a significant impact on your body. It is your responsibility to encourage its production through positive thinking. This simple practice is a powerful way to support your wellness. When your body is healthy, it produces appropriate levels of hormones that help maintain important functions, including metabolism, which is essential for a healthy weight.

Your thoughts generally affect your feelings, and your feelings can influence your habits, especially your choices. These choices can impact your weight management goals. Some people eat when they feel down, and hormones play a role in these behaviors. Choices and thoughts, just like hormones, feed off each other in a continuous loop.

Negative thoughts and feelings can trigger harmful actions in the body. These actions can damage your health. What you think truly matters, even when it comes to your weight management goals. Negative emotions can raise cortisol, the stress hormone, to high levels. Elevated cortisol disrupts blood sugar and other metabolic processes, which often leads to weight gain over time. To maintain a healthy weight, it is important to manage your feelings and emotions well.

Personal Strategies and Faith

People manage their feelings and emotions in many different ways. I have found a strategy that works exceptionally well for me, and it has become an important part of my life. I am always excited to share it with others.

Before I explain further, let me introduce you to my friend. I accepted Jesus Christ as my Savior when I was a preteen. He has changed everything about my life. He is my closest friend, and we are inseparable. His presence has made a huge difference for me. Through every valley and every hill, He has never forsaken me. I submitted my will to Him as a little girl, and it is amazing to see how He has led and continues to guide me. My life would have been very different if I had not accepted Him as my Savior. I have avoided many pitfalls because of His help and guidance. My relationship with Him has given me assurance, both in this life and in the life to come. That is my confidence.

I believe there is life after death. My broad experiences make it impossible for me to change my mind. You may have a different opinion, and that is perfectly okay. Accepting Jesus is a personal choice, and I encourage everyone to make decisions that will affect their life, even after death.

I remember traveling some time ago, wearing a T-shirt with a logo that caught the attention of a man at the airport. He started asking questions, and I had the opportunity to share Christ with him. Without saying much, he told me, "I know there is life after death, and Jesus guarantees eternal life. I have accepted Him." He went on to say that he would rather choose Jesus, even if he found out after death that he was wrong, than risk dying without choosing Jesus and facing hell. I thought that was profound. I smiled and acknowledged his statement with a nod. I will always remember this moment.

Self-Perception and Stewardship

Let's return to the importance of managing your feelings and emotions. Earlier, I discussed your uniqueness and the power of your choices. I often focus on a key scripture that says, "… I am fearfully and wonderfully made"[1]. This thought helps me appreciate my uniqueness, especially when I think about my physical appearance. It reminds me to value my individuality, including how my weight relates to my overall look.

But I don't stop there. I also understand that my body is a temple of the Holy Spirit[2]. Because of this, I strive to care for my body. God needs it here on earth, and that means paying attention to what I put into it. Some of the techniques I've shared help me make good food and lifestyle choices. I use these strategies to ensure I am a good steward of my body.

Good stewardship and a healthy self-perception both influence your weight and self-esteem. That's why I mention them. These two qualities are essential for the motivation and drive needed to achieve and maintain a healthy weight.

You Are at the Center of Your Wellness

Do you realize that all these factors revolve around you? Achieving a healthy weight is not possible without you at the center. What is healthy for you might not be healthy for someone else. Personal health factors matter, and we should all want to feel great. Feeling good affects both your weight and your overall wellness.

Your ideal weight should support your health and wellness. That is what a healthy weight truly looks like. Keep these two factors in mind: weight and wellness. Stay consistent in developing positive habits until they become part of who you are. This consistency will help prevent obsession and frustration with weight changes.

Some people experience extreme swings in their weight, which can lead to an unhealthy focus on managing it. Instead, focus on building the right habits as discussed throughout this book, and your weight will follow. Know and understand your numbers. Stick to the basics. This approach can help you avoid the hype of weight loss trends and give you a strong, effective foundation for the long term. Focus on yourself and your wellness.

Wrap-Up: Key Takeaways

- **Feelings matter in weight management.** Positive emotions support healthy habits and long-term success.
- **Your uniqueness is valuable.** Self-perception influences choices and overall wellness; focus on becoming the best version of yourself.
- **Emotional health impacts BMI.** Worry less, plan more, and take small steps toward your goals.
- **Thoughts affect hormones and habits.** Positive thinking boosts serotonin, while negative emotions raise cortisol, which can lead to weight gain.
- **Manage cravings and stress.** Awareness and intentional choices help break harmful cycles.
- **Faith and mindset can strengthen resilience.** Use strategies that align with your values to stay motivated.
- **Consistency is key.** Build habits that keep YOU at the center of your wellness journey.

Your feelings and thoughts are powerful tools in shaping your health. By managing emotions, practicing positive thinking, and focusing on habits that support your goals, you'll create a lifestyle that promotes both weight and wellness.

Start today, choose thoughts that lift you up and actions that move you forward.

Among the many factors that influence your wellness, hormones play an important role in shaping your feelings. The next chapter will offer tips on how to pay attention to these hormones and use them to improve your mood.

CHAPTER FOURTEEN

Hormonal Balance

Hormones can either help or hinder your weight goals, and the difference often comes down to your daily habits. By understanding what throws them off and what brings them back into balance, you gain a powerful advantage in your wellness journey.

Understand Hormones and Weight Management

Some hormones play a significant role in weight management. To manage your weight effectively, you need to pay attention to these hormones and help them work in your favor. There are also factors that influence these key hormonal regulators of weight loss. By understanding certain basics, you position yourself to overcome hormonal imbalances and promote the health and balance of weight-impacting hormones. Supporting these hormones benefits your entire body.

As you read on, master some foundational strategies to help prevent hormonal imbalances. This is important for both short-term and long-term wellness.

Nutrition and Gut Health

It is essential to eat well-balanced and nutritious foods. Equally important is ensuring that the nutrients from your food are absorbed once they enter your body. Creating conditions in your gut that promote absorption is vital. Many factors affect how well your body absorbs nutrients, but going into excessive detail would take us beyond the scope of this discussion. What you should know is that good bacteria (microflora) in your gut help defend against and can even kill harmful bacteria that enter your body. For a healthy individual, a large number of these beneficial bacteria should be present in the gut. These good gut bacteria have defense mechanisms and also help absorb food, allowing nutrients to reach your bloodstream.

The Impact of Preservatives on Gut Bacteria

Did you know that what you eat can also kill or decrease the number of these good bacteria in your gut? Unfortunately, many people engage in habits that harm these beneficial bacteria. One major culprit is the excessive consumption of preservatives in foods. These good bacteria are essential to your health, so protect them. Preservatives can harm your gut's good bacteria, and many studies support this[1] [2]. For example, a University of Hawaii Maui College study found that food preservatives kill good bacteria in humans[3]. Eating too many preservative-filled foods can do more harm than good. A drop in good gut bacteria can impact food breakdown and may prevent nutrient absorption into your blood. This can affect protein breakdown and absorption, which in turn can harm hormone production. When hormone production is disrupted, the hormones that regulate your eating habits may be affected, impacting your weight management goals. It becomes a cycle.

Making Smart Food Choices

What you eat truly matters. Be watchful and do not take this for granted. Of course, it's okay to enjoy some junk food occasionally. Some wellness ideas I have shared can help you stay in control without overdoing it. If you're interested, try to get a copy of my book, *Healthy Me: Discovering Personal Health and Healing Naturally*. It offers empowering wellness ideas to help you stay on top of your wellness goals.

Preservatives and Hormonal Disruption

Preservatives are a serious enemy to hormone production and balance within the body. Many artificial food additives disrupt hormones like ghrelin and leptin. For example, high fructose corn syrup, when added to foods, can cause leptin resistance[4]. Excessive sugar can have a similar effect, causing the body to ignore "I am full" signals. This can make weight management more challenging. Be aware of these risks.

The Power of Fresh Foods

Eat fresh foods as much as possible. Generally, fresh foods do not contain preservatives. Eating fresh foods most of the time will support your health and help with your weight management.

Long-Term Effects of Preservative-Rich Foods

Excessive consumption of preservative-rich foods can seriously disrupt successful weight management and cause hormonal imbalances. These imbalances can lead to a cycle of cravings for unhealthy foods, as hormonal issues negatively affect your "I am full" cues. This creates a domino effect that influences other body systems over time. Too many preservatives can harm your weight and damage systems that regulate your physical and mental health. Make it a priority to eat fresh foods most of the time.

Wrap-Up: Key Takeaways

- **Hormones matter for weight management.** Ghrelin and leptin regulate hunger and fullness. Imbalances can disrupt progress.
- **Nutrition and gut health are connected.** Good gut bacteria help absorb nutrients and support hormone production.
- **Preservatives harm gut health and hormones.** Excessive preservatives reduce good bacteria and interfere with nutrient absorption, impacting hormone balance.
- **Avoid hormonal disruptors.** Additives like high fructose corn syrup and excessive sugar can cause leptin resistance and increase cravings.

- **Choose fresh foods most of the time.** Fresh, minimally processed foods protect gut health and promote hormonal balance.
- **Limit preservative-rich foods.** Over time, they can trigger cravings, disrupt fullness cues, and harm overall wellness.

Your food choices influence more than your weight; they affect your hormones, digestion, and long-term health. By prioritizing fresh, nutrient-rich meals and limiting preservatives, you'll create a foundation for balance and sustainable weight management.

Start today with one intentional choice: choose fresh over processed. Every small step matters. You've got this!

CHAPTER FIFTEEN

Enhancing Your Digestion

Eating well is only half the story; your body still has to absorb what you eat. With simple, intentional habits, your digestion can help every meal work harder for your health and your weight goals.

The Importance of Absorption

Now is a great time to focus on enhancing absorption. We've established that good absorption is key to hormonal production. It's one thing to eat well, but another for your food to be properly absorbed. For great health, you must pay attention to absorption alongside maintaining a healthy diet. When absorption is effective, every part of your body benefits.

Some people eat nutritious foods but don't promote absorption, which means they miss out on essential nutrients. Poor absorption can lead to hormonal imbalances that negatively impact weight goals, as discussed earlier.

Natural Ways to Promote Healthy Digestion

There are many natural ways to support healthy digestion. One of the best is to chew your food thoroughly. It's easy to overlook this step, but digestion begins in the mouth. Saliva contains key digestive enzymes that help break down the foods you eat.

Saliva is made up of water, electrolytes, mucus, and special cells. It also contains enzymes like amylase and lipase. Amylase breaks down starches into simple sugars your body can use, while lipase breaks down fats into components useful to the body. If you don't chew your food well, it misses out on these enzymes that start digestion. Other parts of the digestive system add more enzymes as food moves through, but it all begins in the mouth.

Here's an idea to help you connect: How do you feel after drinking a smoothie versus chewing the same fruits and veggies? Sometimes, drinking a smoothie can leave you feeling bloated. Gulping it down may prevent it from mixing with saliva, so it misses out on those important enzymes. Fruits have natural sugars, and if the smoothie contains them, amylase in saliva might not begin digestion if gulped down. Amylase helps break down the bonds in complex carbs found in many fruits and veggies. If this initial step of mixing the smoothie with saliva in the mouth is missed, it can lead to bloating and discomfort.

Next time you experience this, try some digestion enhancers. My favorite is ginger, which I like to add to non-dairy fruit and veggie smoothies when the taste is right. There are other options, so experiment to find what works for you. Try to balance eating your fruits and veggies with drinking them in smoothies. Getting the best of both worlds is ideal. Balance is important!

Supporting Gut Health and Absorption

Be mindful of proper digestion and absorption when you eat. Healthy digestion promotes better absorption, helping you enjoy the benefits of your good food choices. We've discussed gut bacteria, their benefits, and the need to reduce preservatives, which can harm and lower your good gut bacteria. Eating well to preserve good gut bacteria is vital for your health. When you protect your gut flora, they help protect your health in return.

Some foods contain good bacteria, such as yogurt and fermented foods. However, food processing can kill some bacteria before they reach your table, so the intended amounts may not always be present. Even people who take probiotics might not get enough good bacteria to the gut, as some may be destroyed along the way. This is why it's important to preserve what you have and make your gut environment suitable for their existence. Select your foods with careful consideration!

Foods and Drinks That Promote Digestion

To support effective digestion, choose foods that naturally promote this process. Foods with moderate to high fiber content are especially beneficial for digestion.

By understanding and applying the food choices we've discussed, you'll gain an advantage for better digestive health.

Sometimes, drinking certain teas or eating specific foods can help your digestion. I share many of these and other health-enhancing features in my book, *Healthy Me*. For example, in most Japanese restaurants, your server will often offer you a cup of green tea after your meal. Green tea is excellent for digestion and also helps burn fat. It offers many other health benefits as well.

Green tea has anti-inflammatory properties and is good for your skin. The next time your server brings you a cup of green tea, don't skip it. And don't let it end there. Try to drink a few cups of green tea each week. This simple habit can support your weight and health goals.

Consider adding some kitchen essentials to your routine: ginger, peppermint, apple cider vinegar, and lemons. These ingredients offer amazing health benefits, much like green tea. Remember to enjoy them in moderation and avoid excesses. Make choices based on your personal preferences, since some natural substances work better for some people than for others. Be patient with the process, try a variety, and see what works best for you. I like to keep a wide selection that works for me and choose from them as needed. You can do the same.

Tailor the amounts to your personal needs, preferences, and body mass. Let natural digestion enhancers support your weight maintenance. There are so many options available. Begin to learn and explore their benefits. Your body benefits most when the foods you eat are properly absorbed into your bloodstream. Proper digestion and absorption are key to reaching your weight and wellness goals. Make thoughtful selections from natural digestion enhancers and use them to your advantage.

Wrap-Up: Key Takeaways

- **Absorption matters.** Eating well is only part of the equation. Your body must absorb nutrients effectively to support health and hormone balance.
- **Chew thoroughly.** Digestion starts in your mouth. Take time to chew so enzymes like amylase and lipase can start doing their job.
- **Balance smoothies and whole foods.** Drinking smoothies too quickly can bypass saliva enzymes, leading to bloating.
- **Support gut health.** Preserve good bacteria by limiting preservatives and choosing foods that promote a healthy gut environment.
- **Add natural digestion enhancers.** Options like ginger, peppermint, green tea, apple cider vinegar, and lemons can aid digestion and overall wellness.
- **Choose fiber-rich foods.** Fiber helps keep digestion smooth and supports fullness, making weight management easier.

Your body benefits most when the food you eat is properly digested and absorbed. By chewing well, protecting gut health, and adding natural digestion boosters, you'll enhance nutrient absorption and support your weight and wellness goals.

Start today with one simple step; chew slowly and savor your food. Every small change adds up to big results over time. You're making progress, and you've got this!

CHAPTER SIXTEEN

Lose It and Keep It Off

Reaching your ideal weight is one thing; learning how to keep it off is where the real transformation happens.

Understanding Your Calorie Needs

You can reach your weight goals by setting clear nutrition goals. Start by knowing the average recommended daily calories for your situation. Calorie needs vary by age, sex, weight, height, and level of physical activity.

It's possible to estimate your daily calorie needs based on your energy requirements. Factors such as sex, age, activity level, height, and weight are important for these estimates. Remember, these are guides, not exact numbers. Generally, boys and men need more calories than girls and women of the same age. Young children usually need between 1,000 and 2,000 calories a day, depending on their sex and activity level. Older children and teens may need 1,400 to 3,200 calories daily, with activity level causing significant differences. Adult women typically need 1,600 to 2,400 calories, while adult men need 2,000 to 3,000 calories. Sedentary people need fewer calories, while very active people need more. Moderately active individuals fall somewhere in between.

At rest, your body uses energy to maintain basic functions like breathing and keeping warm. The number of calories needed for these functions is called your basal metabolic rate (BMR). This is your basic caloric need. Children and adolescents also need energy for growth. Beyond basic needs, daily activities require additional energy, influenced by your height, weight, sex, and activity level. As you age, your resting energy use declines, so you need fewer calories at rest.

Your weight goals, whether you want to lose, gain, or maintain, affect the calories you need each day. Refer to your current weight goal to determine your calorie intake. To estimate your needs, use a reliable online calculator, such as Healthline's[1]. These are estimates, and it's possible to miss a factor unique to you. Use calorie need estimates as a guide, and pay attention to your outcomes. Track your weight trends and how you feel, then make adjustments based on your results. Build healthy habits that suit you, using calorie counts as a guide, aiming for long-term success. Focus on developing lasting habits rather than fixating on calorie counts. Once you master nutrition basics with yourself at the center, proper calorie management will follow naturally. Your body will adjust to hunger cues based on your energy needs, especially if you make smart choices at meals.

Make Your Plate Work for You

Now that you understand calorie needs, use your daily quotas thoughtfully. With practice, you'll master weight management and meet your goals. Your plate, at any meal or snack, is vital to your health. Make it your plate. Own what goes onto it. Choose the components of your plate with care. By making this a regular practice, you can manage your weight and improve your health. These strategies will help you make smart choices and keep eating from becoming a burden.

Strategy #1: Do Not Worry About Food and Calories

Many people worry too much about food and calorie counting, often obsessing over the foods they are "watching." Most do this in an attempt to lose weight. There is a big difference between paying attention and worrying. Your goal should be to pay attention, which leads to planning. Once you make plans, set them aside and execute them as you go, just like any other activity in your life.

Worrying consumes a significant part of your thoughts. You can tell when you're worrying: you get anxious about what to eat, busy counting calories, and fearful of taking a bite of dessert. Food becomes a major focus in your life. You spend too much time planning what to eat and invest resources in foods you believe can magically erase unwanted weight. Unfortunately, worry and its related activities contribute to extreme fluctuations in weight.

Worry can lead to further weight gain, especially if that's not your goal. It can slow digestion and lower metabolism, as your body uses energy to prepare your brain for something it perceives as "scary." Worry activates your body to plan for critical action, even though worrying over food is not the same as being scared. The body treats anxiety in a specific way, and constant worry can have real effects.

Stress raises the hormone cortisol, which increases fat buildup, especially in the stomach, and leads to weight gain. No kind of worry is worth it, especially not about weight and food. Instead, focus on planning what you will eat. Many people make weekly plans. I do, because I have a family and work to juggle. Weekly plans help get everyone involved, and I buy groceries in bulk on shopping days.

Eating is an activity of daily living. Mentally classify it as such. You do this often, as it's vital for survival. Have you ever seen anyone get hungry and pass out or die right away with the initial onset of hunger? I have not seen that happen to an individual with no underlying condition. People with medical conditions should follow their doctor's instructions. If you have no health issues, you can wait until your planned meal when hunger sets in. You can even wait until you prepare what you have planned to eat. Ignoring hunger pangs for a few minutes can help build discipline, which can translate to other parts of your life.

Most food-related worry comes from the question: "What will I do when I get hungry?" Plan and move on. You will cross that bridge safely when you get there, with the plans you have made. Waiting a few minutes between meals is harmless for most people. Hunger pangs will not harm you.

Stop worrying about food and its routines. Even planning for food does not have to be burdensome. Explore meal planning options, and you'll be fine. Keep the strategies you've learned about meal choices in mind when planning. The next strategy will help you address calorie count worries.

Strategy #2: Set Clear Goals and Attain Real Weight Loss

Setting smart goals is important for weight management planning. For many people, weight management is an occasional event, but it doesn't have to be that way, especially if you want to enjoy a healthy you. Weight management can also become an obsession with tasks and weight. Extremes are unsafe and can lead to frequent fluctuations. Find a balance to maintain your ideal weight and reach your health goals. Your health shouldn't suffer for your weight goals; you can enjoy both a healthy weight and a healthy you.

To enjoy this balance, set a clear and SMART weight management goal. For example, aim to lose 3 pounds over the next 30 days. This scenario assumes a goal to lose weight; apply the reverse for a weight gain goal or adjust for weight maintenance.

Set a goal that allows you to stay consistent, since occasional pitfalls, especially at the start, are common. Do not stress or feel discouraged if you stray during your journey. The key is to spot deviations quickly and take action to get back on track. Start with a goal that is realistic. Your goals should always be SMART: Specific, Measurable, Achievable, Relevant, and Time-based.

With these components in mind, losing 3 pounds over the next 30 days is a great example. It is Specific, Measurable, Achievable, Relevant (and realistic), and Time-based.

Weight loss of 1–2 pounds weekly is ideal and considered safe. Keep this in mind to set realistic goals. Our goal of 3 pounds over 30 days assumes a loss of about a pound a week, with consistent progress. This is a good start, and you may even overachieve. Remember to celebrate your achievements.

One pound of body fat may contain between 3,436 and 3,752 calories. Let's use 3,500 calories as a general estimate for one pound of fat. To lose 3 pounds in 30 days, you'll need to cut about 10,500 calories. This is based on the idea that losing one pound requires reducing calories by 3,500. So, for 3 pounds, it's 3 times 3,500.

Now, think about ways to decrease these calories. You can lose about 3,500 calories each week, which could equal a weight loss of 1 pound per week, depending on your body and how it adjusts to burning fat. You can spread the 3,500 calories across the days of the week, decreasing your intake by 500 calories daily over 7 days. This results in 3,500 total decreased calories in a week, a realistic and achievable goal.

To decrease calories by 500 daily, come up with strategies that work for you. This can mean eating a bit less each day and burning calories through exercise. For useful tips on exercise, check out the bonus chapter

"Think Physical Activity" from my book, *Healthy Me: Discovering Personal Health & Healing Naturally*.

To help decide where to cut back calories, keep a food diary for about a month. Observe where you consume most of your calories and identify foods with high calories but little nutritional value, such as sodas, chips, and candies. This will be different for everyone. Start by swapping out soda for water or try carrots instead of chips. Be creative. Also, consider cutting back on food portions. You'll realize how simple it is to decrease your calorie intake. Make it realistic, start with a 250-calorie decrease, and for the other 250, consider exercising to burn those calories. Exercise improves your health and benefits your body's tissues.

This approach is practical, helpful, and realistic for everyday life. It will help you master helpful habits and put you in control of your weight goals. Adjust to fit your preferences so you can maintain your daily 500-calorie cut.

Remember, there is no "one size fits all" formula for weight loss. People's bodies adjust differently during the process. For example, a calorie decrease of 3,500 may lead to a 1-pound loss one week and a 0.5-pound loss another week. At first, most people notice quick weight loss, then the pace slows as the body adjusts. Keep this in mind and don't get discouraged if progress slows. Maintain consistency and find joy in your progress. Different body systems burn fat in distinct ways, and your body is unique. Take time to understand your body and make choices that fit you best.

Using this strategy, set your personal goal, write down your plan, and you'll be on your way to success.

Wrap-Up: Key Takeaways

- **Know your calorie needs.** Use reliable tools to estimate daily requirements based on age, sex, weight, height, and activity level.
- **Focus on habits, not obsession.** Pay attention to food choices and planning without worrying or overthinking calories.
- **Set SMART goals.** Make them Specific, Measurable, Achievable, Relevant, and Time-based for realistic progress.
- **Aim for safe weight loss.** A reduction of 1–2 pounds per week is ideal; plan gradual calorie cuts and pair them with exercise.
- **Track and adjust.** Use a food diary to identify high-calorie, low-nutrient foods and replace them with healthier options.
- **Celebrate progress.** Stay consistent, avoid discouragement, and enjoy the journey toward lasting habits.

Your success in weight management comes from planning wisely and practicing consistency, not from stress or extremes. Start today by setting one realistic goal and creating a simple plan to achieve it. Every small step counts, and your progress will add up over time.

You've got this!

CHAPTER SEVENTEEN

Essential Factors

There's always more behind a number on the scale. When you understand what truly influences your journey, you can focus on the choices that move YOU forward.

Many people focus on their weight as just a number. While numbers are important, there are other factors that influence those numbers. It's essential to understand these factors and how they affect your weight goals.

Looking Beyond the Numbers: Genetics

BMI is an important measure and often the most relatable number. It is unique to everyone, as it considers your height in relation to your body mass.

When it comes to body fat and its distribution, your genetic makeup plays a key role. Genetics influence your body shape and determine how your body stores fat. They also affect certain aspects of hormonal production that impact weight management. Environmental factors, such as your food choices and activities, interact with your genetics and influence how your body produces hormones and stores fat.

You may not have control over your genetic makeup, but you do have control over your everyday choices. This is where you can make a real difference. Your choices matter; they can magnify or diminish the effects of your genetics. The important thing is that you get to make your own choices, and those choices should be worth it. Pay attention to the decisions you make.

Choices and Environment: What You Can Control

While you can't change your genes, your choices can influence how they affect you. Your environment, which includes your daily decisions, can have a significant impact. Certain genes can even change (mutate) over time, often due to environmental factors and lifestyle choices. These changes can be positive or negative, depending on the choices made. Never underestimate the power of your decisions; they can have a lasting impact, even across generations. Make the best choices for yourself.

Genetic factors matter, but environmental factors can impact genetics. Your choices matter. Once you feel confident about your choices from earlier chapters, focus on building a healthy YOU. Don't let comparisons to others distract you. Your body fat distribution is unique, so embrace your appearance with confidence. You have a special genetic makeup. For example, look at your wrist bone and compare it to someone else's. Bone structure varies in size, and your wrist size gives an indication of your body frame. Everyone's genetic makeup is different, and this is important to consider when managing your weight.

Age, Metabolism, and Nutrition

Age can affect how quickly your body breaks down food and turns it into energy (metabolism). Metabolism determines the amount of energy (calories) your body uses to maintain itself. Kids and teens gain fat at different times as they grow, so it's important to focus on their nutritional needs and habits rather than just body fat. This is especially important for teenagers, particularly girls, since boys and girls differ in how fat is distributed in their bodies. Genetics play a key role in this process.

Talk to your kids as they grow. Help them build habits that allow them to take charge of their nutrition and weight goals. This will help them avoid comparing themselves to others and obsessing over weight. Teach them how to be the best version of themselves. This will boost their confidence as their bodies change.

As you grow older, your metabolism slows down. The rate at which you break down food decreases by about 10 percent each decade after age 20. This is another reason why calorie needs vary with age. Don't expect to burn energy at the same rate as you did in your teenage years. You may not need as many calories as you did then, depending on your current activity level. Refer to your earlier calorie needs estimation to see how this applies to you.

Embrace Your Unique Journey

Keep track of your calorie needs and use them to support good nutrition for a healthy YOU. Genetics also affect metabolism. Some people burn calories faster than others and tend to lose fat more quickly due to a higher metabolic rate. Their metabolism works in their favor for weight loss. This group usually loses weight faster when they plan.

Some people feel discouraged about managing their weight, often comparing themselves to others. This can lead to unrealistic expectations and extreme weight loss measures, which may deprive them of important nutrition and harm their health over time. Play it safe and focus on yourself.

You are unique and different from everyone else. Keep these factors in mind and remember to focus on YOU as you work toward your weight management goals. Avoid comparisons and learn more about yourself. Take key principles from this book to guide you as you discover more about yourself. Master habits that put you in charge and allow you to maintain a healthy weight for the long run.

Wrap-Up: Key Takeaways

- **Weight is more than a number.** Genetics, environment, age, metabolism, and daily choices all influence your journey.
- **Genetics matter, but choices matter more.** You can't change your genes, but you can make decisions that support your health and work with your genetic blueprint.

- **Lifestyle and environment shape outcomes.** Your daily habits can amplify or reduce genetic tendencies and even impact future generations.
- **Metabolism changes with age.** Calorie needs decrease over time, so adjust your nutrition and activity accordingly.
- **Support kids and teens.** Teach them healthy habits and confidence to prevent comparison and obsession with weight.
- **Focus on YOU.** Avoid comparing yourself to others. Embrace your uniqueness and build habits that fit your life.

Your weight journey is personal. By understanding the factors that influence it and making intentional choices, you'll create a plan that works for YOU. Stay consistent, trust the process, and celebrate every step forward.

You've got this!

CHAPTER EIGHTEEN

Key Numbers for a Healthier YOU

Your numbers tell a story, but they don't define you. Key numbers can guide you, but your uniqueness gives them meaning.

It's important to consider numbers in context. Always put yourself and your unique factors at the center of any analysis. Once that's clear, remember that numbers play a big role in many parts of life, just as they do in finances. Keeping an eye on key numbers is important for successful goal management, and your weight is no exception.

There are three critical numbers to keep in mind when it comes to your weight and wellness: your BMI, waist circumference, and waist-to-hip ratio. These numbers will revolve around you when you understand yourself and your wellness goals. They can help you pay attention to key aspects of your health as they relate to your weight.

Understanding Your BMI

From our previous discussions, you know the role of your BMI and how it can help you determine when you are in a good place with your weight goals. While BMI has its limitations, it is generally a safe and simple number to pay attention to when managing your weight. Take an interest not only in your weight but also in your overall health as it relates to your weight. That is a key focus of this book.

Waist Circumference: A Simple, Powerful Measure

Other key numbers and measurements show how your weight relates to your health. Waist circumference is a very important number. It gives a good indication of the amount of fat accumulation around organs in the body. Think about the various organs close to your waistline. Organs need the right amount of fat around them for protection, but your goal is to avoid excess. Too much fat can lead to high levels of free fatty acids (triglycerides) in the blood, which lab tests can detect. Excessive fat can put you at risk for conditions that result from obesity, such as heart disease and type 2 diabetes. Focus on maintaining good health while also managing your weight goals.

Measuring your waist circumference is easy and can be done at home without risk or expensive tools. To get started, grab a tape measure and stand upright. Find your natural waistline, usually located above your waistline and below your ribcage; the narrowest part of your body's trunk. To locate it more easily, try bending to your side; the crease that forms is a spot on your natural waistline.

Once you've found your natural waistline, wrap the tape measure around your waist as you would when wearing a belt. Keep the tape horizontal and close-fitting, but do not apply excessive pressure. Take note of the measurement immediately after you breathe out. That will be your waist circumference. You can check as often as you choose. Women who are not pregnant should aim for a waist circumference of 35 inches or less[1]. For men, 40 inches or less[2]. These are general recommendations. As with anything, some people may have measurements that are outliers; for them, those may be their safe, normal measurements.

If your numbers fall outside the standard, discuss it with your physician. They can look at your situation and suggest ways to help you stay safe, especially if you have a condition that limits your physical activity. Generally, maintaining a healthy weight is a great place to start. Many people notice their waist size getting smaller when they reach a healthy weight.

Waist-to-Hip Ratio: Understanding Fat Distribution

The waist-to-hip ratio is another helpful measurement to consider. This ratio shows an individual's health based on fat distribution. It reflects how fat is distributed within the body and is worth noting. Since you know your waist measurement, you can also measure your hips to understand the ratio better.

To measure your hips, wrap the tape around the widest part of your hips, usually where your buttocks stick out the most. Ensure the tape remains horizontal and note the measurement, using the same unit as your waist measurement (inches or centimeters). To get your waist-to-hip ratio, divide your waist measurement by your hip measurement.

The World Health Organization recommends a healthy range of 0.9 or less for men and 0.85 or less for women[3]. Exceeding these numbers increases the risk of heart and metabolic issues. Keeping this ratio below 0.85 for men and 0.75 for women is ideal.

Wrap-Up: Key Takeaways

- **Know your key numbers.** BMI, waist circumference, and waist-to-hip ratio are important indicators of health and weight status.
- **BMI is a helpful guide.** Use it as a simple tool to monitor your weight, while remembering its limitations.
- **Measure your waist.** Aim for 35 inches or less for women and 40 inches or less for men to reduce health risks.
- **Check your waist-to-hip ratio.** Keep it below 0.9 for men and 0.85 for women for better heart and metabolic health.
- **Use numbers as guides, not stressors.** They are tools to help you make informed decisions, not reasons to worry.

Your numbers tell part of your health story, but they don't define you. Use them as helpful markers to guide your choices and track progress. Start today by measuring your waist and hips. You will gain valuable insight into your wellness journey.

Stay focused, stay positive, and keep moving toward your goals. You've got this!

CHAPTER NINETEEN

Diet Plans and Medications: Do They Work? Do I Need Them?

Every diet and medication promises results, but your long-term success depends on the habits underneath.

Many people choose diet plans for weight loss and management. While following a diet plan can be helpful, without a strong foundation, it can become a struggle. Rapid weight fluctuations can be frustrating, especially when you notice sharp ups and downs. Knowing what influences your weight and how to control it can save you from frustration. Keep the concepts you are learning here and use them to your benefit.

Are you on a special diet for weight loss or management? Have you ever been somewhere and couldn't find an option for your dietary plan? What did you do? Stayed hungry or ended your program? What you are about to learn will help you navigate such issues with confidence.

Are you currently on any diet plan? If so, which one? I am often asked which diet plan is best, and my answer is always the same: diet plans tend to be trendy, and most people go along with the trends. Many jump on trends and find quick success, but often struggle to achieve long-term weight management. Revolve diet trends around you, not the other way around. Make adjustments to fit your needs while aiming for lasting success.

Your success with diets depends on what you know about food groups. Understanding how they impact your weight goals is key. This knowledge will help you adjust your approach and set you up for long-term success. Being able to make adjustments frees you from the stress of feeling stuck in a diet plan. It allows you to enjoy the journey, regardless of which diet trend you choose. To see real, lasting success, position yourself at the center of diet plans and trends. Consider your personal preferences, allergies, or medical restrictions with certain foods. Always focus on YOU with any health plan, including diet plans.

The truth is, no diet plan or weight-loss trick will support you for the long run, unless it's part of a healthy, sustainable weight-management lifestyle that puts YOU at the center. Even after bariatric surgery to reduce stomach size, some people discover that their stomachs can gradually readjust when old habits remain unchanged. As mentioned earlier in the book, stomach muscles can stretch and adapt over time based on how much food you regularly eat. That's why the real focus has to be on you. Build the right habits, mindset, and choices. Not quick fixes. Quick fixes may feel good in the moment, but lasting change comes from commitment and a focus on right habits. The concepts you've learned from this book empowers you to succeed.

You've learned how food groups can impact your weight loss or management goals. Apply this knowledge to support your goals and make smart food choices to avoid pitfalls in any diet trend. Also, know that certain diets may not be suitable for everyone. Talk to your doctor before starting any diet, especially if you've had surgery or a health issue.

Think of any diet or weight loss trend, and you will realize that using concepts from this book puts you ahead and in charge to succeed. I will review a few popular diet trends and connect them to ideas we've discussed earlier in this book. This approach will help you see the bigger picture and relate new information to what you already know. By making these connections, you'll be better equipped to succeed with any diet trend you choose. Remember, you are free to select what works best for you. If you decide to follow a diet, it should support your weight goals, not make them harder to achieve.

The Atkins and Paleo Diets

The late Dr. Robert Atkins[1] popularized the Atkins Diet in 1992 with his book, *Dr. Atkins' New Diet Revolution*. His research dates back to the 1960s.

The Atkins Diet is all about low carbohydrates and high protein and fats. It usually begins with cutting carbs and boosting protein and fat intake. It also promotes eating high-fiber foods, which appeals to some vegans. When the body has few carbohydrates, it starts to burn fat for energy, promoting weight loss.

People have chosen this diet for various reasons, including potential health benefits and enjoyment of the foods promoted. Some healthcare professionals have suggested it to patients. Over time, the Atkins trend made room for other evolving diets.

Dr. Loren Cordain helped popularize the Paleo Diet, which is designed to mimic the eating habits of our ancient hunter-gatherer ancestors[2]. When you think of "hunter-gatherers," protein comes to mind, which connects the Paleo Diet to the Atkins Diet in some ways. Hunters relied on meat and wild plant foods, so the Paleo Diet also includes nuts and other plant-based options. The creators of this diet believe that our ancestors thrived on these foods and lived healthier, longer lives as a result.

Some people still follow the Atkins Diet, while others have switched to the Keto Diet, which we will review soon.

The Atkins Diet continues to be popular, even as new dietary trends emerge. As you observe these evolving trends, keep in mind that many share important features you've already learned, whether or not they are labeled as a specific dietary plan. By sticking to proven scientific principles, you'll make sound choices. Earlier in this book, you learned key tips about selecting foods based on food groups, and you'll see more connections and pointers as you read along.

Before starting any diet, especially weight-loss plans, consult with your healthcare provider. This is especially important if you have any health conditions, as some diet plans may not be suitable for everyone.

Let's pause for a moment of reflection and self-review. From our earlier discussions, consider the role protein plays in weight loss and management. How important is it? You can revisit previous sections about food groups and your choices to check your understanding. Reflect on these answers. They are meant to guide you in selecting the right foods for your meals. The Atkins diet focuses on the potential benefits of protein intake. However, it is possible to go overboard without looking at your overall health. As we move forward, keep in mind the connection between protein and the dietary plans we're discussing.

It's possible to have the right foundation in place, which you now have. As trends change, take time to understand them. Focus on food choices that support your weight management goals. This approach will position you for personal success, no matter how trends evolve. Diets may come and go, but the habits you form with solid knowledge will last.

Effective, lasting habits are built on a strong foundation of knowledge. There is one food group that remains constant, regardless of dietary trends; vegetables. Including vegetables in your plate selections is a key essential you've mastered. With this foundation, YOU are at the center, not the diet trend. Dietary choices should revolve around you.

To give you an overview, the Atkins Diet has about four phases[3]. The first phase, called the Induction Phase, begins with extreme carbohydrate limitation and progresses through the other phases. The diet encourages drinking at least eight glasses of water daily, eating more vegetables, and limiting fruit because of sugar. It also emphasizes maintaining intake of proteins and healthy fats.

The final phase is lifetime maintenance, where the dieter is expected to have learned the key parts of the diet and is ready to maintain the benefits gained. The Atkins Diet has evolved over time to address drawbacks that some people experience. Remember, the focus of this book is YOU, tailoring choices to best suit your weight management goals. More people could benefit from the Atkins Diet if they learned how to adjust their choices, such as knowing the right amount of protein for their weight and avoiding excess.

Consuming too much protein can strain the kidneys, especially for those with kidney issues. Healthy kidneys filter out waste from protein digestion, but some people's kidneys may struggle. Eating too much animal protein can cause related byproducts of its digestion to build up in the blood, which may lead to other health issues.

Even for healthy individuals, excessive protein intake can cause problems. It's important to consume regular amounts of protein. Uric acid, a major byproduct of protein breakdown, can accumulate if not eliminated efficiently, potentially leading to gout and other issues. Eating too much animal protein can trigger flare-ups or worsen gout for those who are prone to it.

During the peak popularity of the Atkins Diet, there was also an increase in gout cases. Could there have been a correlation? Use what you've learned to make your own inferences. Some trends offer clues to potential pitfalls.

Learn from them and move forward. Avoid adopting diet plans for quick results if they could harm your long-term health. Remember my wellness concept of Balance and adjust your choices to fit your needs and include a variety of foods. This will help you avoid potential pitfalls, even if you choose a diet plan like Atkins.

You can maximize any diet without experiencing negative effects. Most people notice immediate weight loss when starting the Atkins Diet because it is designed to stimulate fat burn. I encourage you to consider how this diet fits your long-term health goals. Look into possible downsides, then decide what is best for you. You might find it helpful to try the diet for a short time and then make adjustments that suit your long-term goals. What you've learned will help you make good choices and decisions. Keep your food group selections centered around YOU. Do not eat less protein than your body needs, but avoid excess. Eating enough protein will help you maintain your weight management goals.

Pair your proteins with healthy fats, complex carbohydrates, and plenty of vegetables and fruits. This will help you feel full and support your goals. You can adjust a diet plan like Atkins to fit your personal needs, helping you build lasting habits. These habits will guide you in making good choices, no matter what options you face.

The Keto Diet

The Keto Diet, or Ketogenic Diet, centers on eating a high amount of fat, with low carbohydrates and adequate protein. Originally developed in the 1920s, it was used to help treat epilepsy in children before anticonvulsant medications became more common.

When you eat carbohydrates, your body converts them into glucose, which is used for energy. Your brain also relies on glucose for its activity. If you eat very few carbs, your body still needs energy, so it begins to burn fat instead. The liver then turns this fat into fatty acids and ketone bodies. When ketone bodies build up in the blood, the body enters a state called ketosis.

Some children with epilepsy have fewer seizures when their blood has higher levels of ketones, which is why the ketogenic diet was originally developed. In 1921, Dr. Russell Wilder at the Mayo Clinic coined the term "ketogenic diet"[5] for this purpose. Today, the Keto Diet is a popular trend, and many people have found benefits from it.

If you are considering a diet, always put yourself first. Examine the plan in detail to ensure it fits both your short-term weight loss goals and your long-term health needs. There are many variations of the Keto Diet, and like most diets, it may not be suitable for everyone. It is important to discuss your options with your physician, especially if you have any health conditions or a relevant medical history. Focus on your long-term health, safety, and wellness in every decision, especially when managing your weight.

Some research suggests the Keto Diet may offer health benefits beyond weight loss, but not everyone will experience these benefits. Remember, a diet with enough protein and moderate fat will help you feel full longer. Add complex carbohydrates, plenty of vegetables, and some fruits to your meals. This slows digestion and helps keep hunger at bay. By focusing on the four main parts of your plate, you'll feel fuller longer and boost your overall wellness. Balance your intake of carbohydrates, proteins, and fats to avoid excess. Eat a variety of foods for better health, and choose more plant-based options when possible.

If you're not allergic to any plant foods and your medications don't interact with them, include a variety of plant foods in your diet. Most vegetables are low in calories and add health-boosting substances to your bloodstream. Stick to plant-based complex carbs like corn and potatoes. The closer your food choices are to the farm, the better for your health. Eat fresh and complex, and choose the right amounts of carbs for yourself. Reviewing the food choices chapter often will help you make the best decisions.

Using these tips, you can customize a Keto Diet that suits you, supporting both short-term and long-term goals. Like most diets, many people see weight loss benefits when they start the Keto Diet, along with other associated benefits. Before starting any weight-loss diet, ask yourself: "How will this affect my long-term health?" Not considering this question at the start could have consequences later.

The Keto Diet can pose risks for some people, such as those with fat metabolism disorders, liver issues, or pancreatitis. Always talk to your doctor before starting a Keto Diet, as it could cause complications. Check your health condition and have conversations with your healthcare providers before making any changes.

Do not put your health at risk in pursuit of weight loss. Weight loss and long-term health should go hand in hand, with YOU at the center. Asking yourself personal questions can help you decide how long to stay on a diet, even at the start. This can also help you jumpstart a weight loss plan if that is right for you. Once you begin a diet plan, try to build routines that help you develop healthy habits. These habits will help you reach your weight management goals and maintain your desired weight while supporting overall wellness.

You've learned to make smart food choices, which will help you stay on track with your health and wellness goals. You've also gained tips to help you decide if a diet plan is right for you. If you choose not to follow a specific dietary plan, you can still do well with all you have learned.

Be aware of the risks associated with diet trends and avoid excess. Diabetic Ketoacidosis (DKA) is a rare condition that occurs more frequently in people with type 1 diabetes, and sometimes in those with type 2 diabetes. DKA can happen when there is not enough insulin, often triggered by illness, stress, or poor diet. In DKA, blood sugar remains in the bloodstream and cannot enter the body's tissues for storage or energy use. Without insulin, the body begins to break down fat for energy, releasing large amounts of ketone bodies.

Diabetic ketoacidosis can be life-threatening, causing acidic body fluids, dehydration, and organ damage. Ketogenic diets produce only small amounts of ketones, which is different from ketoacidosis. Small amounts of ketones cause a state called ketosis, which is not the same as ketoacidosis. Both involve burning fat and creating ketone bodies, but it is important to keep their differences in mind.

I mention ketoacidosis because people often ask about DKA. It's important to understand it. A common question is, "Can someone on a keto diet make too many ketones?" I usually say that I haven't seen studies showing that healthy people on a ketogenic diet produce harmful ketone levels, but I always stress the importance of staying cautious. The body can do surprising things, even things it has never done before. There can always be a first time, and other problems can trigger these moments. It's better not to be that rare statistic.

We will learn more about the long-term effects of the Ketogenic Diet in the coming years, just as we did with the Atkins Diet. Potential consequences of excess fat consumption are worth watching. Pay attention to how too many ketone bodies might affect long-term health, similar to issues caused by too much uric acid from high-protein diets like Atkins. Watch out for organs that break down excess fat, such as the liver. Over time, potential problems could especially affect these organs. Some people may face new health issues we do not know about yet, as organs become overwhelmed by excess byproducts of fat metabolism. We may not know all the risks now, so stay cautious and maintain balance.

Focus on building healthy habits. Daily choices can impact long-term health, and seeing how today's decisions shape your future is important. Take charge of your choices today. Stick to safe zones and avoid eating too much of anything, even healthy foods, especially with diet trends. Adjust your diet to match your long-term wellness goals, whether you choose the Keto Diet or another plan. Avoid becoming a victim of negative statistics related to shifting dietary trends. Use the tips discussed, stay in control, and keep yourself at the center of your choices. Enjoy your freedom and focus on long-term health, no matter what dietary plan you choose.

Popular Weight Loss Medications: GLP-1

The use of medications for weight loss has become a growing trend. Glucagon-like peptide-1 (GLP-1) agonist medications, often called GLP-1 meds, have gained popularity for their role in supporting weight loss. These medications work by mimicking the action of a naturally occurring hormone in the body.

GLP-1 is produced in the gut after we eat and helps regulate blood sugar levels. It supports the body in secreting insulin, slows down digestion, and increases the feeling of fullness between meals. While I won't go into extensive detail about GLP-1 and its related medications, my goal is to highlight how the concepts discussed in this book relate to the way GLP-1 meds work.

Most people first learned about GLP-1 medications as treatments for type 2 diabetes. Examples include Ozempic and Trulicity. More recently, these medications have received attention for their use in weight loss.

Some people need medications to help them lose weight, and doctors may recommend them based on individual conditions or risk factors. Even in these cases, it's important to put measures in place to sustain weight loss for the long term. That's why everyone can benefit from the concepts in this book. The strategies you've learned will help you manage your weight for the long run, without getting lost in the latest trends.

Every weight loss trend connects in some way to the Essential Trio discussed: Satiety (the feeling of fullness), Speed (the rate of digestion), and Snacking (limiting snacks between meals). Your food choices and habits can help you stay in shape, and every weight loss trend, including the use of GLP-1 meds, tries to manage an aspect of this trio.

Some people lose weight with trends or medications but regain it when they stop. Building sustainable habits is the key to successful weight management, and you now have the tools to do so.

It's also important to note that there isn't enough data yet to show the long-term effects of some of these trends, including medications. More information becomes available as more people use them, and unfortunately, some negative effects may only become clear over time. It's always better to be safe than sorry. Be careful, build the right habits, take care of yourself holistically, and enjoy a good quality of life. Stick with a healthy approach to weight management that keeps YOU at the center. Use the concepts you've learned from this book to manage your weight and your health effectively.

Wrap-Up: Key Takeaways

- **Diet plans can help, but habits matter most.** Your long-term success depends on building a strong foundation of healthy routines.

- **Trendy diets like Atkins, Paleo, and Keto offer short-term results without the right habits.** Always put yourself at the center; adjust plans to fit your health, preferences, and goals.
- **Balance your plate.** Include protein, healthy fats, complex carbs, and plenty of vegetables for sustainable wellness.
- **Consult your doctor before starting any diet or medication.** Safety comes first, especially if you have health conditions.
- **Moderation is key.** Avoid extremes with protein or fat intake to prevent health issues like kidney strain or gout.
- **Weight loss medications, such as GLP-1 agonists, may help some people.** Remember, habits and not medications, are the foundation for lasting success.
- **Focus on the Essential Trio: Satiety, Speed, and Snacking.** These principles apply to every diet trend and medication strategy.
- **Your long-term health should always be the priority.** Avoid quick fixes and build habits that support balance and wellness.

Diets and medications can play a role, but they are not magic solutions. Your success comes from consistent, intentional choices that fit your life and protect your health. Start today by focusing on balance and building habits that last.

You've got this!

CHAPTER TWENTY

Think Physical Activity

You don't need a gym membership to change your health; you just need to move. When you start thinking in terms of "physical activity" rather than "exercise," you open the door to powerful, everyday progress.

This information comes from my previous book, *Healthy Me: Discovering Personal Health & Healing Naturally.*

Physical activity plays a crucial role in healthy weight management. When you find creative ways to fit movement into your daily schedule, you can achieve amazing results.

Little steps truly count! Often, when people think about physical activity, they picture scheduled exercise. While that's part of it, physical activity goes far beyond planned workouts. For many, exercise means a set routine, maybe an hour at the gym. That's wonderful, and seeing others persevere can motivate us all. If you enjoy going to the gym, and it fits your life, keep it up!

At certain times in life, when demands are lighter, it's easier to make time for scheduled exercise, including trips to the gym. But as a busy working mother with a busy husband, children, and social commitments, I know that even finding time to drive to the gym twice a week can be a real challenge. Balancing family, work, and social life takes skill and patience.

Juggling your own schedule alongside those of your loved ones can take up much of your day, making it hard to fit in everything you want to do. Often, gym time is the first thing to go when responsibilities increase. As parents, we may choose to take our kids to their activities rather than go to the gym ourselves. That's a natural choice, and you should never feel guilty for making it.

To complicate things, many of us are exhausted by the end of the day, physically or mentally, from work and other demands. In those moments, the last place we want to be is at the gym. Sometimes, we just want to relax and watch TV, which can even add to our mental stress.

For many, this pattern can continue all week. It can become even more discouraging when we feel guilty about missing the gym. Some people begin to associate missing gym sessions with an inability to exercise, and eventually give up on movement altogether when their plans are disrupted.

This is where it's important to pause and reflect. Have you considered how much your loved ones want you to stay healthy for as long as possible? They count on you to help them reach their next milestones. All the effort you put into supporting them, whether it's working to pay the bills or helping with their activities, means they need you for the long haul. Taking care of yourself isn't just about you; it's also a gift to those you care about. When you prioritize your health, you're better able to support the people who matter most in your life.

Think physical activity! This mindset can help you stay creative and help you reap the benefits of exercise, even when your plans for the gym don't work out. For example, planning and engaging in family activities like walking, bike riding, or jogging can be enjoyable and rewarding for everyone. You can still gain the benefits of a scheduled exercise routine by incorporating other forms of physical activity that fit easily into your daily schedule. This approach is especially useful on days when you can't make it to the gym.

Physical activity is simply any movement that uses energy. At home, this could mean going up and down the stairs, mowing the lawn, playing and running around with your kids in the backyard, swimming, walking, or jogging in your neighborhood. There are many options. Choose what works for you.

Staying physically active allows you to tailor movement to your tolerance and daily routine. This includes all forms of exercise, but keeping this concept in mind makes it easier, more enjoyable, and more doable. Even walking up the stairs at work for five minutes instead of using the elevator counts as physical activity.

Personally, focusing on physical activity helps me stay motivated and creative. It encourages me to be active throughout my day and to enjoy the same benefits as scheduled exercise. Keeping this concept in mind can help you purposefully add movement to your day.

Remember, physical activity can be moderate or vigorous. The Centers for Disease Control and Prevention (CDC) recommend adults get at least 150 minutes of moderate aerobic activity, or 75 minutes of vigorous aerobic activity, or a combination each week[1]. As a guideline, moderate activity means you breathe deeper and harder than when you're at rest. You should be able to talk, but not sing a song without pausing for breath. You'll usually start sweating a few minutes into moderate activity, such as brisk walking or mowing the lawn.

Vigorous activity means your heart is working at its maximum, and your breathing is even deeper and harder. Talking or singing becomes difficult, and you'll need to pause frequently to catch your breath. You'll break into a sweat much quicker than with moderate activity. Examples include jogging, biking, or hiking in hilly areas.

If you haven't been physically active for a while, start slowly. It's important to consult your healthcare provider if you have any activity restrictions, as may be with some heart conditions. Your provider can help you determine what levels of physical activity are safe for you.

Physical activity offers many outstanding benefits beyond strengthening muscles. For heart health, imagine your arteries as straws or water hoses. Over time, fatty deposits like cholesterol can build up and narrow these arteries, blocking blood flow and increasing the risk of heart problems. Exercise increases blood flow pressure, which can help clear away these deposits, much like water pressure clearing debris from a hose.

When we exercise, it's similar to increasing the water pressure in a hose. This increased blood flow can help prevent or decrease the buildup of plaques in our arteries, much like water pressure clearing away debris from the walls of a hose or straw. If you stick with regular physical activity, this simple analogy highlights one way exercise can improve your heart health.

Physical activity offers a wide variety of "aerobic" exercises if you stay creative. Aerobic activity is especially important because it's all about oxygenation, making oxygen available to your body's tissues. Here's where being physically active ties directly into building your immune health: oxygen, oxygen, oxygen. Let movement help deliver oxygen to your tissues. Oxygen is essential for your body's function, helping cells produce energy efficiently. Think of how oxygen fuels a fire to burn brighter, and connect that to how it can help your body feel more energized. You could eat all the right foods, but if your body doesn't get enough oxygen, it won't be able to produce energy at its best.

Without diving into the details of cellular energy production, remember this: oxygen acts as fuel for your body's energy. Next time you've eaten well but still feel tired, try exercising and notice the difference in how you feel.

My love for biology always brings me back to cellular connections, and here I use concepts from microbiology. Most bacteria, viruses, and fungi cannot survive or thrive in an oxygen-rich environment. These organisms do better without oxygen and are called anaerobes. This is important to remember as we talk about oxygen's role in the body. Boosting oxygen supply to your tissues can help your immune system by creating an environment where many harmful pathogens struggle to survive.

There are advances in therapy that use our understanding of oxygen's role in immune health, including treatments for autoimmune diseases. One example is Hyperbaric Oxygen Therapy (HBOT). HBOT is under active research, and many studies show it can be effective for treating autoimmune diseases in certain people[2]. In HBOT, individuals receive 100% oxygen in a pressurized chamber, which enhances the body's ability to heal itself[3]. HBOT is often used alongside other treatments.

Studies have shown that different levels of oxygen can influence the severity of inflammation and how well anti-inflammatory medications work[4]. Higher oxygen levels have shown more positive results compared to lower levels. HBOT further demonstrates how the body can respond better to certain medications when you take those small steps to improve oxygen availability to your cells through physical activity.

I share all of this to encourage you: you can boost your body's ability to heal and maintain good health by strengthening your immune system through physical activity. In my experience as a nurse, one of our main focuses, even for patients recovering from surgery, is to help them engage in physical activity at a level they can tolerate, always considering any restrictions based on their condition or diagnosis. We encourage even the smallest amount of movement when possible. The benefits are too important to overlook. Every cell and tissue in your body, from your gut to your brain, benefits from physical activity.

Physical activity, among its many other advantages, makes oxygen more available to your tissues and supports your immune health. I keep emphasizing "physical activity" because every little step truly counts. While the gym can be helpful, you don't have to wait for a gym session to benefit from movement. Personally, I've found that setting 10-minute goals for physical activity throughout my day helps me stay consistent. Whether it's during a lunch break walk or a fun activity, these short bursts add up. This approach is easier to fit into a busy schedule and helps me avoid feeling guilty when I can't carve out longer periods for exercise. Even on busy days, I feel reassured knowing that my five- and ten-minute sessions contribute to my health goals.

Physical activity also stimulates the release of "feel-good hormones" called endorphins, which bring many health benefits. Your mental health and emotions can improve with regular movement. In fact, people with anxiety disorders often see symptom improvement from exercise[5]. Endorphins make a significant difference in our mental well-being.

I remember a time when I faced health challenges. When I was able to get out of bed, even short walks around the house, no matter how brief, helped me feel better mentally and emotionally. I highly recommend staying physically active, even if it's just a little each day. Every bit is better than doing nothing. Pause and think about small ways you can get moving during your day. Then, make a plan to put those ideas into action and boost your immune health. Your body will thank you.

Wrap-Up: Key Takeaways

- **Physical activity is essential for weight management and overall health.** You don't always need long gym sessions; small, consistent steps count.
- **Find creative ways to move.** Walking, climbing stairs, playing with kids, or short bursts of activity throughout the day all make a difference.
- **Start where you are.** Even five or ten minutes of movement can boost your health and energy.
- **Follow recommended guidelines.** Aim for a minimum of 150 minutes of moderate activity or 75 minutes of vigorous activity weekly, adjusting for your health and lifestyle.
- **Movement benefits your whole body.** It supports heart health, improves oxygen delivery, strengthens immunity, and enhances mental well-being.
- **Celebrate progress, not perfection.** Every effort matters. Focus on consistency and enjoy the benefits of staying active.

Your body thrives on movement. Whether it's a brisk walk, a few minutes of stretching, or playful time with family, every step brings you closer to better health. Start today with one small action. Your future self will thank you.

You've got this!

End Note

Healthy Weight: Simple Strategies for Successful Weight Management** is more than a book. It's a guide to building a lifestyle that works for you. The principles you've learned here are designed to help you create balance, confidence, and habits that last.

Remember, weight management is not about perfection. It's about progress, consistency, and making choices that support your health and happiness. Every small step matters.

At the time of publishing this book, there is new guidance on the food pyramid. This book was written before that guidance was released, yet you will notice how empowering these concepts are. When you focus on the core concepts in this book, you set yourself up for success with your weight and wellness goals, no matter how recommendations or trends continue to change around you.

Revisit the wrap-up sections whenever you need a quick refresher, and keep applying the strategies that fit your life. Celebrate your wins, learn from challenges, and stay focused on your long-term goals.

Your journey to a healthier, happier YOU starts now, and you have everything you need to succeed.

Take control.
Build habits that last.
Enjoy the freedom of living well.

References

Chapter 2

1. Hamwi, G. J. (1964). *Therapy: Changing dietary concepts.* American Diabetes Association.
2. Robinson, J. D., Lupkiewicz, S. M., Palenik, L., Lopez, L. M., & Ariet, M. (1983). Determination of ideal body weight for drug dosage calculations. *American Journal of Hospital Pharmacy, 40*(6), 1016–1019.
3. Peterson, C. M., Thomas, D. M., Blackburn, G. L., & Heymsfield, S. B. (2016). Universal equation for estimating ideal body weight and body weight at any BMI. *The American Journal of Clinical Nutrition, 103*(5), 1197–1203. https://doi.org/10.3945/ajcn.115.121178
4. Hirche, T. O., Hirche, H., Jungblut, S., Stern, M., Wagner, T. O., Wiedemann, B., & German CFQA Group. (2009). Statistical limitations of percent ideal body weight as measure for nutritional failure in patients with cystic fibrosis. *Journal of Cystic Fibrosis, 8*(4), 238–244. https://doi.org/10.1016/j.jcf.2009.03.004
5. ScyMed. (n.d.). Ideal body weight (Hamwi method). Retrieved December 20, 2022, from http://www.scymed.com/en/smnxpn/pndfc237.htm

6. Centers for Disease Control and Prevention. (n.d.). Adult BMI calculator. Retrieved December 20, 2022, from https://www.cdc.gov/healthyweight/assessing/bmi/adult_bmi/english_bmi_calculator/bmi_calculator.html
7. Centers for Disease Control and Prevention. (n.d.). Children and teens BMI calculator. Retrieved December 20, 2022, from https://www.cdc.gov/healthyweight/bmi/calculator.html
8. Centers for Disease Control and Prevention. (n.d.). Adult BMI calculator. Retrieved December 20, 2022, from https://www.cdc.gov/healthyweight/assessing/bmi/adult_bmi/english_bmi_calculator/bmi_calculator.html

Chapter 3

1. Centers for Disease Control and Prevention. (n.d.). Adult BMI calculator. Retrieved December 20, 2022, from https://www.cdc.gov/healthyweight/assessing/bmi/adult_bmi/english_bmi_calculator/bmi_calculator.html
2. Centers for Disease Control and Prevention. (n.d.). About adult BMI. Healthy Weight. Retrieved December 20, 2022, from https://www.cdc.gov/healthyweight/assessing/bmi/adult_bmi/index.html#interpretedAdults
3. Centers for Disease Control and Prevention. (n.d.). Losing weight. Retrieved December 20, 2022, from https://www.cdc.gov/healthyweight/losing_weight/

Chapter 5

1. Naik, S., Bhide, V., Babhulkar, A., Mahalle, N., Parab, S., Thakre, R., & Kulkarni, M. (2013). Daily milk intake improves vitamin B-12 status in young vegetarian Indians: An intervention trial. *Nutrition Journal, 12*, 136. https://doi.org/10.1186/1475-2891-12-136
2. National Institutes of Health. (n.d.). Office of dietary supplements – Vitamin B12. Retrieved December 20, 2022, from https://ods.od.nih.gov/factsheets/VitaminB12-HealthProfessional/
3. Davoodi, S. H., Shahbazi, R., Esmaeili, S., Sohrabvandi, S., Mortazavian, A., Jazayeri, S., & Taslimi, A. (2016). Health-related aspects of milk proteins. *Iranian Journal of Pharmaceutical Research, 15*(3), 573–591.
4. Pinnock, C. B., Graham, N. M., Mylvaganam, A., & Douglas, R. M. (1990). Relationship between milk intake and mucus production in adult volunteers challenged with rhinovirus-2. *The American Review of Respiratory Disease, 141*(2), 352–356. https://doi.org/10.1164/ajrccm/141.2.352

Chapter 8

1. Longmatey, Y. (2019). *Healthy me: Discovering personal health and healing naturally* (p. 272).
2. Longmatey, Y. (2019). *Healthy me: Discovering personal health and healing naturally.*
3. Longmatey, Y. (2019). *Healthy me: Discovering personal health and healing naturally.*

Chapter 11

1. Klok, M. D., Jakobsdottir, S., & Drent, M. L. (2007). The role of leptin and ghrelin in the regulation of food intake and body weight in humans: A review. *Obesity Reviews, 8*(1), 21–34. https://doi.org/10.1111/j.1467-789X.2006.00270.x
2. Biggers, A. (n.d.). Hunger pangs (pains): 7 causes and how to alleviate them. *Medical News Today*. Retrieved December 20, 2022, from https://www.medicalnewstoday.com/articles/321725.php#causes
3. Klok, M. D., Jakobsdottir, S., & Drent, M. L. (2007). The role of leptin and ghrelin in the regulation of food intake and body weight in humans: A review. *Obesity Reviews, 8*(1), 21–34. https://doi.org/10.1111/j.1467-789X.2006.00270.x
4. Longmatey, Y. (2019). *Healthy me: Discovering personal health and healing naturally.*

Chapter 13

1. *The Holy Bible, New King James Version.* (n.d.). Psalm 139:14.
2. *The Holy Bible, New King James Version.* (n.d.). 1 Corinthians 6:19.

Chapter 14

1. University of Hawai'i Maui College. (n.d.). Food preservatives kill beneficial bacteria found in humans. Retrieved February 11, 2022, from

https://maui.hawaii.edu/studentaffairs/uh-maui-college-research-finds-that-food-preservatives-kill-beneficial-bacteria-found-in-humans/

2. Hrncirova, L., Machova, V., Trckova, E., Krejsek, J., & Hrncir, T. (2019). Food preservatives induce Proteobacteria dysbiosis in human-microbiota associated Nod2-deficient mice. *Microorganisms*, 7(10), 383. https://doi.org/10.3390/microorganisms7100383
3. University of Hawai'i Maui College. (n.d.). Food preservatives kill beneficial bacteria found in humans. Retrieved February 11, 2022, from https://maui.hawaii.edu/studentaffairs/uh-maui-college-research-finds-that-food-preservatives-kill-beneficial-bacteria-found-in-humans/
4. Shapiro, A., Mu, W., Roncal, C., Cheng, K. Y., Johnson, R. J., & Scarpace, P. J. (2008). Fructose-induced leptin resistance exacerbates weight gain in response to subsequent high-fat feeding. *American Journal of Physiology: Regulatory, Integrative and Comparative Physiology, 295*(5), R1370–R1375. https://doi.org/10.1152/ajpregu.00195.2008

Chapter 16

1. Gunnars, K. (2019, December 20). How many calories should you eat per day to lose weight? *Healthline*. Retrieved December 20, 2022, from https://www.healthline.com/nutrition/how-many-calories-per-day#calorie-calculator

Chapter 18

1. Centers for Disease Control and Prevention. (n.d.). Waist circumference. Retrieved December 20, 2022, from https://www.cdc.gov/healthyweight/assessing/index.html
2. Centers for Disease Control and Prevention. (n.d.). Waist circumference. Retrieved December 20, 2022, from https://www.cdc.gov/healthyweight/assessing/index.html
3. World Health Organization. (2011). *Waist circumference and waist-hip ratio: Report of a WHO expert consultation*. Geneva, Switzerland.

Chapter 19

1. CNN. (2003, April 17). Diet guru Dr. Robert Atkins dead at 72. Retrieved December 20, 2022, from http://www.cnn.com/2003/HEALTH/04/17/obit.atkins/
2. The Paleo Diet®. (n.d.). Easy paleo recipes, nutritional science & more! Retrieved December 20, 2022, from https://thepaleodiet.com/
3. Atkins. (n.d.). Low carb diet program and weight loss plan. Retrieved December 20, 2022, from https://www.atkins.com/
4. Wheless, J. W. (2008). History of the ketogenic diet. *Epilepsia, 49*(Suppl 8), 3–5. https://doi.org/10.1111/j.1528-1167.2008.01821.x
5. Wheless, J. W. (2008). History of the ketogenic diet. *Epilepsia, 49*(Suppl 8), 3–5. https://doi.org/10.1111/j.1528-1167.2008.01821.x

Chapter 20

1. Centers for Disease Control and Prevention. (2018). Physical activity. Retrieved from https://www.cdc.gov/physicalactivity/basics/adults/
2. Saito, K., Tanaka, Y., Ota, T., Eto, S., & Yamashita, U. (1991). Suppressive effect of hyperbaric oxygenation on immune responses of normal and autoimmune mice. *Clinical and Experimental Immunology, 86*(2), 322–327.
3. Harch Hyperbaric Oxygen Therapy. (2018). Retrieved May 11, 2018, from http://www.hbot.com
4. Federation of American Societies for Experimental Biology. (2013, December 2). Oxygen levels affect effectiveness of anti-inflammatory therapies. *Science Daily*. Retrieved March 11, 2018, from http://www.sciencedaily.com/releases/2013/12/131202121536.htm
5. DeBoer, L. B., Powers, M. B., Utschig, A. C., Otto, M. W., & Smits, J. A. (2012). Exploring exercise as an avenue for the treatment of anxiety disorders. *Expert Review of Neurotherapeutics, 12*(8), 1011–1022. https://doi.org/10.1586/ern.12.73

Acknowledgements

I'd like to express immense gratitude to my father in heaven for bringing these great concepts to light through me.

To my amazing husband Daniel and our precious children Jezniel and Josiah, whose unwavering love and support challenge me to make a difference in the lives of others each day, I say thank you.

To my dad, the late Dr. A. O. C. Nettey-Marbell (1936-2017) and my mom, Mrs. Beatrice Nettey-Marbell, I'm forever grateful for your love, support, the many opportunities that have stirred within me a lifelong love for health and wellness. And to my amazing siblings, your families, and my friends, I am grateful for each one of you!

To my clients, thank you for motivating me to impact more lives in the area of health and wellness. Continue to take charge and live well!

www.ingramcontent.com/pod-product-compliance
Lightning Source LLC
LaVergne TN
LVHW022212200926
848481LV00006B/1942